The "I Have a Life"

Pregnancy Guide

Get Ready for Your New Life—
Without Losing Your Old One

edited by Andrea Mattei

Adams Media
Avon, Massachusetts

Published by Adams Media, an F+W
Publications Company
57 Littlefield Street
Avon, MA 02322
www.adamsmedia.com

ISBN: 1-59337-594-8
Printed in the United States of America.

J I H G F E D C B A

**Library of Congress Cataloging
in Publication Data**
The "I have a life" pregnancy guide / edited
by Andrea Mattei.
p.   cm.
ISBN 1-59337-594-8
1. Pregnancy. 2. Self-care, Health.
I. Mattei, Andrea.
RG525.P74 2006
618.2   dc22
2006005206

*This book is available at quantity discounts
for bulk purchases. For information, please
call 1-800-872-5627.*

This publication is designed to provide accurate and
authoritative information with regard to the subject
matter covered. It is sold with the understanding
that the publisher is not engaged in rendering legal,
accounting, or other professional advice. If legal
advice or other expert assistance is required, the services of a competent professional person should be
sought.

—From a *Declaration of Principles* jointly
adopted by a Committee of the American
Bar Association and a Committee of
Publishers and Associations

Many of the designations used by manufacturers
and sellers to distinguish their products are claimed
as trademarks. Where those designations appear in
this book and Adams Media was aware of a trade-
mark claim, the designations have been printed with
initial capital letters.

Contains portions of material adapted and abridged
from *The Everything® Pregnancy Book, 2nd Edition* by
Paula Ford-Martin, ©2003, F+W Publications, Inc.;
The Everything Pregnancy Organizer by Margueriet
Smolen, ©2000, F+W Publications, Inc.; and *The
Everything® Pregnancy Fitness Book* by Robin Elise
Weiss, ©2004, F+W Publications, Inc.

The "I Have a Life" Pregnancy Guide is intended as a
reference volume only, not as a medical manual. In
light of the complex, individual, and specific nature
of health problems, this book is not intended to
replace professional medical advice. The ideas, procedures, and suggestions in this book are intended
to supplement, not replace, the advice of a trained
medical professional. Consult your physician before
adopting the suggestions in this book. The author
and publisher disclaim any liability arising directly
or indirectly from the use of this book.

Contents

Part 3: Getting Down to Other Business / 115

Introduction

*W*hether you are pregnant or just thinking about having a baby, your life is about to change. But it's still *your* life, and this one-stop guide will help it stay that way!

If you are overwhelmed by the sheer volume of pregnancy and childbirth information available and are just too busy to read thousands upon thousands of pages, *The "I Have a Life" Pregnancy Guide* is just what you need. It covers everything you need to know to have a healthy and safe pregnancy in a quick, easy-to-understand way that fits in with your busy lifestyle. You thought you were busy *before* you got pregnant—imagine how your life will be now that you have to deal with everything from doctor's appointments to diapers and nutrition to nursing!

Have no fear—from the positive pregnancy test to postpregnancy weight loss, this guide doesn't leave anything out. Each chapter highlights important tasks for each stage so you can break down your extensive to-do list into manageable pieces.

Your body has a to-do list of its own. To learn what it's up to, you can read all about how your body is changing at each stage of your pregnancy, and how your baby is developing every month. And you'll be getting loads of tests at all those doctor's appointments you have to go to—check out Chapter 5 to know what each and every one of those needles and blood tests is for.

Of course, your baby's health is your biggest concern for the next nine months. But what about you? Check out Chapter 8 for sound advice on what to eat and what *not* to eat. To stay healthy, you'll also need to stay fit, so look for special exercises for each month of your pregnancy.

Everyone knows that with pregnancy comes some amount of discomfort. Throughout the book, you'll find quick and easy tricks for easing those little (okay, maybe not so little) aches and pains associated with each stage of your pregnancy—swollen ankles, heartburn, headaches, backaches, morning sickness. . . .

Besides taking good care of your growing baby and your (also growing) self, you'll need to figure out the best place to deliver your baby. The days of women being limited to their local hospital are gone—and we'll explore all your options. Plus, you'll develop a personalized birthplan—an essential aspect of labor and delivery.

Then, after the big day has come and gone, what do you do with that perfect little smiling (okay, wailing) newborn? From breastfeeding basics to career concerns, this guide leaves no room for guessing. We've got you covered.

In the meantime, try to relax, de-stress, and take it one day at a time. After all, you're becoming a mom! You should start to get to know that little person growing inside you and take time to savor your pregnancy. Nine months may seem like a long time, but it'll go by in the blink of an eye. . . .

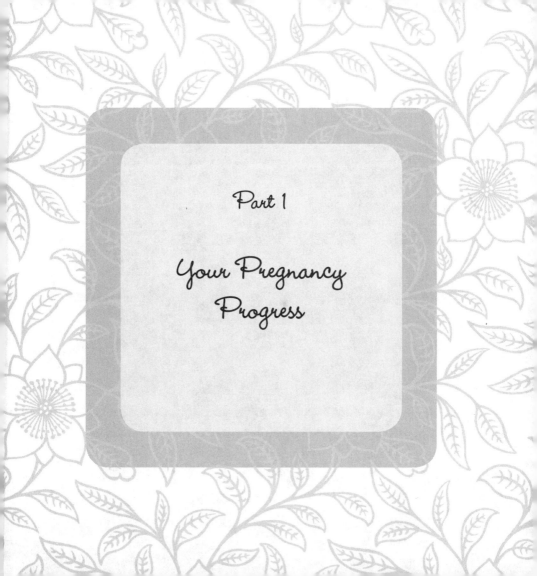

Part 1

Your Pregnancy
Progress

Chapter 1

So You're Pregnant: The First Trimester

During the first trimester of pregnancy, your body is hard at work forming one of the most intricate and complex works of nature. By the end of your first official month of pregnancy, your developing child will have grown an astonishing 10,000 times in size since fertilization.

The First Month

this month's priorities

Congratulations are in order! At last—you've dreamed of becoming pregnant, and now, you're pretty sure you are. To confirm the good news, you'll want to:

- ○ Buy a pregnancy test kit, and test yourself at home.
- ○ Write down your symptoms.
- ○ Find a doctor.
- ○ Make an appointment to get examined.

Baby This Month

Your developing baby (called a zygote) travels from the fallopian tube and into the uterus (or womb). After fertilization, the zygote begins a process of rapid cell division, and by day four it has formed a small solid cluster of cells known as a morula. The morula finishes the trip down the fallopian tube, reaching the uterus about three to four days after fertilization.

The Blastocyst

By day five or six, your baby takes on its third name change in less than one week as the morula grows to a blastocyst. The blastocyst contains two distinct cell layers with a cavity at the center. The inner layer will evolve into the embryo, and the outer layer will develop into the placental membranes—the amnion and the chorion. Within days, the blastocyst nestles into the nutrient-rich lining of your uterus (the endometrium) as implantation begins about one week after conception. Wispy fingers of tissue from the chorion layer called chorionic villi will anchor the blastocyst to your uterine wall where they will begin to build a network of blood vessels. These villi are the start of the placenta, a spongy oval-shaped structure that will "feed" the fetus (via the umbilical cord) with maternal nutrients and oxygen throughout pregnancy.

The Embryo

About fifteen days after conception, the blastocyst officially becomes an embryo. Next to the embryo floats the yolk sac, a cluster of blood vessels that provide blood for the embryo at this early stage until the placenta takes over. The embryo is surrounded by a water-tight sac called the amnion (or amniotic sac). The amniotic fluid that fills the sac provides a warm and weightless environment for your developing baby. It also serves as a sort of embryo airbag, protecting baby from the bumps of your daily routine. Nature efficiently double bags your baby, surrounding the embryo and the amnion with a second membrane called the chorion.

··············· **need to know** ·······················

During this first four weeks of development, your embryo has laid the groundwork for most of its major organ systems.

As month one draws to a close, baby's heart is beating, lung buds have appeared, and construction of the gastrointestinal system and liver are well underway. The neural tube, the basis of the baby's central nervous system, has developed and the forebrain, midbrain, and hindbrain are defined. He (or she) is starting to look more like a person, too. The first layer of skin has appeared, facial features are surfacing, and arm and leg buds are visible. It's an amazing list of accomplishments considering your baby is about the size of a raisin (less than ¼ inch long).

Your Body Changes

At this point in your pregnancy, you might not notice any significant changes in your shape and size. Although you aren't menstruating, you feel slightly bloated and your breasts may also start to increase in size. The areolas around your nipples may enlarge and darken and your breasts will most likely be tender in pregnancy (although a supportive sports bra can help). You may also experience increased vaginal secretions similar to those you get premenstrually. These typically last throughout pregnancy and may actually worsen in the third trimester. Normal vaginal secretions in pregnancy are clear to white in color, mucuslike, and both odor and pain free. If you experience discharge that is thick, foul-smelling, off-color, or accompanied by itching, blood, or pain, contact your health care provider immediately to rule out infection or other problems.

What You Feel Like

Building a baby is hard work, and even though it's early in the process, it isn't unusual to feel tired and run down right now. If at all possible, try to grab a nap during the day and make early bedtime a priority. You may also find yourself spending more and more time in the bathroom. You are urinating more frequently due to high levels of progesterone, which relax your bladder muscles. Unfortunately, frequent urination is one symptom that will likely remain with you throughout pregnancy as your baby grows and the uterus exerts more and more pressure on your bladder. Constipation may become a problem due to increased levels of progesterone; you also may experience problems if you're taking iron supplements. Your cardiovascular system is undergoing big changes right now as it adjusts to meet baby's growing demand for the oxygen and nutrients your blood is carrying. Circulating pregnancy hormones dilate, or expand your blood vessels to accommodate an eventual 50 percent increase in blood volume. Your cardiac output, a measurement of how hard your heart is working to pump blood, increases by 30 to 50 percent, while your blood pressure drops. This is why you may find yourself feeling faint.

:·························· **need to know** ························:

If you are dizzy or lightheaded, sit or lay down on your side as soon as possible.

Try not to lay flat on your back, particularly later in pregnancy as the pressure your uterus places on both the aorta and the inferior vena cava (two of the large blood vessels that help keep oxygen circulating to you and baby) will actually make the dizziness worse.

And then, there's the most notorious of all pregnancy symptoms—morning sickness. Referred to by clinicians as nausea and vomiting of pregnancy (NVP), up to 80 percent of women experience one or both of these symptoms at some point in their pregnancy.

NVP Remedies and Safety

The following treatments have been associated with some success in lessening symptoms of NVP in clinical trials. **Speak with your health care provider before adding any new supplements to your diet.**

Ginger. Ginger snaps and other foods and teas that contain ginger may be helpful in settling your stomach.

Acupressure wristbands (Sea-Bands). Sometimes used to ward off motion and sea-sickness, these wristbands place pressure on what is called the P6, or Nei-Kuan, acupressure point. Available at most drugstores, they are an inexpensive and noninvasive way to treat NVP.

Vitamin B and B6. Thiamine (B1) and B6. These supplements have reduced NVP symptoms in several clinical trials. It has been suggested that NVP is a sign of B vitamin deficiency.

Other treatments that women report as helpful include:

Eating smaller, more frequent meals. An empty stomach produces acid that can make you feel worse. Low blood sugar causes nausea as well.

Choosing proteins and complex carbohydrates. Protein-rich foods (e.g., yogurt, beans) and complex carbs (e.g., baked potato, whole grain breads) are good for the two of you and may calm your stomach.

Eat what you like. Most pregnant women have at least one food aversion. The better foods look and taste, the more likely they are to stay down.

Drink plenty of fluids. Don't get dehydrated. If you're vomiting, you need to replace those lost fluids. Some women report better tolerance of beverages if they are taken between meals rather than with them. Turned off by water and juice right now? Try juicy fruits like watermelon and grapes instead.

Brush regularly. Keeping your mouth fresh can cut down on the excess saliva that plagues some pregnant women.

Talk to your provider about switching prenatal vitamins. If it makes you sick just to look at your vitamin, perhaps a chewable or other formulation will help. Iron is tough on the stomach, so your provider might also recommend a supplement with a lower or extended release amount.

At the Doctor

Set up your first prenatal care visit as soon as you know you are pregnant. For now through the seventh month, you'll be seeing your provider on a monthly basis. If you're seeing a new doctor or midwife, expect your initial visit to be a bit longer than subsequent checkups since you'll be asked to fill out medical history forms and insurance paperwork.

Your provider will ask plenty of questions about your health history and the pregnancy symptoms you have been experiencing. Make sure that you take advantage of this initial appointment to ask about issues that are on your mind as well. In addition to this interview time, you will undergo a thorough physical examination, give a urine sample, and have blood drawn for routine lab work. Your provider will probably supply you with educational brochures and pamphlets on prenatal care, nutrition, office policies, and other important issues. Start a folder or notebook for keeping pregnancy information together, and store it near your bed or other favorite reading and relaxation spot for easy access. Add a pad of paper to your "pregnancy portfolio" so you can jot down any questions for your provider. Call your doctor immediately if you experience any of the following symptoms:

- Abdominal pain and/or cramping
- Fluid or blood leaking from the vagina
- Abnormal vaginal discharge
- Painful urination
- Severe headache
- Impaired vision (e.g., spots, blurring)
- Fever over 100.4 degrees Fahrenheit or chills
- Excessive swelling of face and/or body
- Severe and unrelenting vomiting and/or diarrhea

You should also become familiar with the signs of preterm labor. While a good dose of common sense should be used in contacting your doctor after hours, in most cases "better safe than sorry" applies. Remember, your provider works for you, and you're heading up this pregnancy team. If something just doesn't feel right to you, make the call.

The Second Month

- ○ Read about your unborn baby.
- ○ Continue to record your symptoms.
- ○ Learn Kegel exercises.
- ○ Learn how to nap.
- ○ Look at your clothes and start planning for your maternity wardrobe.

Baby This Month

Your unborn child has now advanced to about ½ inch in length. By the end of the month, he or she will be about one inch long. The tail she was sporting disappears around week eight, and her closed eyes start to move from the sides of the head to their permanent location. The face is further defined by a nose and jaw, and the buds of twenty tiny baby teeth are present in the gums by week ten. The palate and vocal cords also form around this time.

Important organ systems are nearly completed by the end of month two. The right and left hemispheres of your baby's brain are fully formed and brain cell mass grows rapidly. Soft bones begin to develop, and the liver starts to manufacture red blood cells until the bone marrow can take

11

over the job in the third trimester. Your unborn baby is also giving his brand new organs a workout. Heart chambers form, the pancreas begins to produce insulin, and the liver secretes bile. The stomach produces gastric juices while the intestines, which have developed in the umbilical cord, move up into the abdomen by the end of the month. Floating in about 1.5 ounces of amniotic fluid, your baby has plenty of room for flexing the muscles she is now developing. At about eighteen to twenty weeks, when the second trimester is in full swing and her quarters become a bit closer, you will feel the first flutterings, known as quickening.

Your Body Changes

Even though you may not have put on any additional weight yet, your growing uterus is pushing the boundaries of your waistline. On average, most women gain between 2.5 to 5 pounds in the first trimester. Changes in skin and hair are common in pregnancy.

·················· **pregnancy treat** ··················

Hair that was fine and thin may become thick and shiny during pregnancy, and that fabled pregnancy "glow" may actually be your flawless, blemish-free complexion.

On the other end of the spectrum, acne problems and hair breakage and thinning may occur. Chloasma, also known as melasma, may cause a masklike darkening or lightening of your facial skin. Freckles and moles are prone to darkening, as well as other pigmented areas of your skin (e.g., areolas). To minimize chloasma and other hyperpigmentation, use a good sunscreen (SPF 30 or higher) to cover exposed skin when you're out in the sun. Your gums may start to bleed when you brush your teeth, a condition known as pregnancy gingivitis. Be sure to floss and brush regularly to keep your teeth and gums healthy. A warm saltwater rinse may soothe swollen gum tissues (ask your doctor first if you have a history of high blood pressure). Now is a good time to schedule a thorough cleaning with your dentist; in a few months, leaning back in a dental chair will be uncomfortable, if not impossible.

What You Feel Like

The stomach rumblings of the first month continue, and an increase in nausea and vomiting may actually occur as hCG levels peak toward the end of this month. On the plus side, your NVP may start to get better in the coming weeks as hCG levels wane. If you're one of those lucky women who do not experience morning sickness at all, you're probably not escaping the feelings of fatigue. Take the hint your body is giving you and take time out to rest.

At the Doctor

If you had your preliminary appointment last month, your prenatal office visits will now start to slip into a routine. At a minimum, expect to step on the scale, give a urine sample, and have your blood pressure checked at the start of each appointment. You'll also be asked about any new or continuing pregnancy symptoms, and your provider will feel the outside of your abdomen to determine the size of your uterus.

Get the Most Out of Monthly Checkups

Bring along that list of questions that have come up since your last visit. Again, write these down when they come to you and your partner so you won't have to rely on your memory in the doctor's office. Make sure your questions are answered before you leave. Stop her before she leaves the exam room and let her know you have a few questions.

Never feel like you're being pushy or overbearing (remember, you're leading this team).

Mood Swings

If you're normally the even-keeled type, the emotional outbursts that often accompany pregnancy can be downright alarming. You aren't losing control or losing your mind, you're experiencing the normal mood swings of pregnancy. Although this emotional liability may continue throughout pregnancy, it is typically strongest in the first trimester as you adjust to hormonal and other changes. Given the transformation your body is going through and the accompanying aches and pains, you have every right to be cranky. Of course, no one is happy when that happens, so take steps now to reduce your stress level and achieve some balance.

Stress and Stress Management

It's easy to get stressed out over what may seem like an overwhelming amount of preparation for your new family member. Your body is already working overtime on the development of your child; try to keep your commitments and activities at a reasonable level to prevent mental and physical overload.

Added psychological stress can make the discomforts of pregnancy last longer and feel more severe. Anxiety may also impact your child's health. An increase of corticotropin-releasing hormone (CRH), a stress-related substance produced by the brain and the placenta, has been linked to preterm labor and low birth weight. Research has also suggested a possible connection between first-trimester maternal stress and congenital malformations. As you rush to get everything "just so," remember that your little one is not going to care if the crib matches the dresser, but he will feel the effects of your excess tension.

Effective stress management involves finding the right technique for you. Relaxation and meditation techniques (e.g., progressive muscle relaxation, yoga with your doctor's consent), adjustments to your work or social schedule, or carving out an hour of "me" time each evening to decompress are all ways you can lighten your load. Exercise is also a great stress control method, but be sure to get your doctor's approval regarding the level of exercise that is appropriate for you.

The Third Month

this month's priorities

- ○ Talk about tests with your doctor.
- ○ Evaluate your medicine cabinet.
- ○ Go bra shopping.
- ○ Consider telling people your good news.

Baby This Month

By the end of this month, baby will grow to over three inches in length and almost one ounce. If you could look at his face, you'd see that his ears and closed eyelids have now fully developed. His head accounts for one-third of his total length, and his tongue, salivary glands, and taste buds have also formed.

He is now getting all of his nutrients through the fully formed placenta, an organ that you and your fetus share. The umbilical cord tethers the fetus to the placenta, which provides it with nutrients and oxygen and transports waste materials away. Your baby's heart is pumping about twenty-five quarts of blood each day, and a lattice of blood vessels can be seen through his translucent skin, which is starting to develop a coat of fine downy hair called lanugo. His, or her, gender is apparent since the external sex organs have now fully differentiated, but it will take a combination of luck and technical skill for an ultrasound operator to reveal if you have a son or daughter.

Your Body Changes

Your uterus is about the size of a softball and stretches to just about your pubic bone. Weight gain will pick up in the second trimester and peak in the third as your baby starts to fill out your womb. Don't take the "eating for two" cliché literally—300 extra calories per day is about all you'll require to meet your baby's nutritional needs. Gaining too much can exacerbate the aches and pains of pregnancy, place an extra strain on your back, and may put you at risk for hypertension (high blood pressure) problems.

At the same time, if you find the aversions and nausea of pregnancy have you only keeping down a certain type of not-so-nutritious food, don't feel bad about it. The most important thing right now is keeping food down and your energy up. Try experimenting with some healthier variations of your favorite food if your stomach will take it, and hang in there. By the end of the first trimester most women report that their morning sickness gets better or completely disappears. While twenty-five to thirty-five pounds is the average suggested total weight gain for a pregnancy, your height and build will influence that number.

······················ **need to know** ······················

If your provider hasn't mentioned a weight goal for your pregnancy, ask him what his expectations are.

Most important, don't let the scale become an obsession. Focus instead on the quality of food you're eating and on getting some regular exercise (cleared with your provider first). Your health, and baby's health, is the ultimate goal of this pregnancy.

What You Feel Like

Although nausea and vomiting may finally be waning thanks to a decline in hCG levels, constipation, gas, and occasional heartburn may take over as the gastrointestinal pests of the next trimester. Constipation is caused by an increase in progesterone, which can act to slow down the digestive system. Later in the pregnancy, pressure on the intestine caused by your growing uterus adds to the problem. Iron supplements or prenatal vitamins with added iron can also cause constipation, so talking to your provider about the possibility of a dosage adjustment or an extended release formula may be in order. An increase in dietary fiber, plenty of water intake, and exercise as approved by your health care provider may also help to get things going again. Be sure to consult your doctor before taking any stool softeners or laxatives. Gas may become a source of discomfort and occasional embarrassment as well. Consider cutting back on foods that worsen the problem (e.g., onions, beans, broccoli, cabbage, carbonated drinks). Fiber you take to eliminate constipation can also aggravate gas problems. Try small, frequent snacks instead of large meals to keep the burps at bay. Other pregnancy symptoms that may continue or begin this month include:

- Fatigue
- Headaches
- Frequent urination
- Increased saliva

- Tender breasts
- Nasal congestion and/or runny nose
- Nausea
- Occasional dizziness or faintness

At the Doctor

Make sure your husband or partner makes this month's prenatal appointment. You're both in for a treat as you begin to experience the sights and sounds of your growing child.

Baby's Heartbeat

Hearing the steady "woosh-woosh" of your baby's heart for the first time is one of the most thrilling and emotional moments of pregnancy. Your chance at first contact happens this month as your provider checks for the fetal heartbeat using a small ultrasound device called a Doppler or

Doptone. If you have a retroverted uterus (also known as a tipped or tilted uterus), it's possible the Doppler won't detect the heartbeat just yet. Don't be alarmed; by your next prenatal appointment you will probably be able to hear her loud and clear.

Forgetfulness

Lost your car keys for the fifth time this week? Like any mom-to-be, you've got a lot on your mind. That alone may have you forgetting what used to be second nature and misplacing things. Although researchers have looked at the problem of memory impairment in pregnancy, there hasn't been a clear consensus on what the definitive cause is. Pregnancy hormones, sleep deprivation, and stress have all been suggested as possible culprits. A 2002 study published in the *Journal of Reproductive Medicine* found that women in their second trimester of pregnancy who reported memory problems had lower blood levels of the neurotransmitters norepinephrine, epinephrine, and serotonin than their nonpregnant peers, suggesting that these brain chemicals may somehow be related to memory loss. Whatever the cause, forgetting appointments and misplacing things can leave you feeling muddled and helpless. Try relying less on your memory by writing notes, sticking to a routine, and living by a written or electronic organizer. If you aren't the Palm Pilot type, start requesting a twenty-four-hour advance phone call reminder when you schedule service appointments such as an in-home appliance repair or a salon appointment. Having a system—whatever it is—is the key to staying reasonably organized and mentally together during this hectic time.

Chapter 2

Energy Kick: The Second Trimester

*W*elcome to the second trimester, or what many women consider "the fun part." Your energy is up, and your meals are staying down. You and your baby are headed into a period of rapid growth now, so hang on and enjoy the ride. Here's a look at what you can look forward to in month four.

The Fourth Month

this month's priorities

○ Review tests with your practitioner.
○ Schedule test dates.

Baby This Month

Snoozing, stretching, swallowing, and even thumb-sucking, your fetus is busy this month as he tests out his new reflexes and abilities. He is losing his top-heavy look as his height starts to catch up to his head size. By the end of this month, he will measure about six to eight inches in length and weigh approximately six ounces.

He has grown eyebrows, eyelashes, and possibly even a little hair up on top. The long bones of his arms and legs are growing as cartilage is replaced with spongy, woven soft bone in a process called ossification. Skeletal development will continue long after birth and well into adolescence and young adulthood. Your baby is inhaling and exhaling amniotic fluid, practicing his technique for his first breath in the outside world. The lungs are already generating cellular fluid and a substance known as surfactant.

The placenta is approximately three inches in diameter this month, and the attached umbilical cord is about as long as the fetus and continues to grow. Fetal blood is being pumped through this little body at about four miles an hour, exiting through two large arteries in the umbilical cord and on to the placenta. In the placenta, baby's waste products (urine and carbon dioxide) are exchanged for oxygenated, nutrient-rich blood that is returned to the fetus via an umbilical cord vein.

Your Body Changes

If you weren't showing last month, chances are you will have a definite pregnant profile by the end of this month. Your uterus is about the size of a head of cabbage, and its top tip lies just below your belly button.

What You Feel Like

Your appetite may start to pick up this month. You'll need a healthy craving or two to fuel fetal growth—about 60 percent of your total pregnancy weight (about eleven to fifteen pounds) will be gained in this trimester. Heartburn may start to become a persistent problem as your uterus crowds your stomach and the smooth muscles of your digestive tract remain relaxed from the hormone progesterone. Some tips for putting out the fire:

- Avoid greasy, fatty, and spicy foods.
- Avoid alcohol and caffeinated drinks (e.g., cola, tea, coffee); these relax the valve between the stomach and the esophagus and exacerbate heartburn.
- Keep a food log to try to determine what your heartburn triggers are.
- Eat smaller, more frequent meals instead of three large ones.
- Drink plenty of water between meals to reduce stomach acid.
- Don't eat just before you go to bed or lay down to rest.
- Pile pillows on the bed to assist gravity in easing heartburn while you sleep.

If heartburn symptoms won't relent, there are several over-the-counter antacids and medications available that are considered safe to use in pregnancy. Speak with your doctor to find out which one may be right for you.

As if heartburn wasn't enough to deal with, pregnancy may start to become a real pain in the rear, literally. Many women develop hemorrhoids, which are caused by increased pressure on the rectal veins secondary to pregnancy. By straining to have a bowel movement, you put stress on the rectal veins, which can become blocked, trapping blood, turning itchy, painful, and perhaps even protruding from the anus. Exercise, a high-fiber diet, and plenty of water can help to avoid constipation and straining with bowel movements that may aggravate the condition. Try easing the pain with an ice pack, a soak in a warm tub, wipes with witch hazel pads, or a topical prescription cream as recommended by your doctor. Be sure to speak with your provider about hemorrhoids if they do occur. While they typically resolve after pregnancy, in some cases clotting occurs, and surgery is necessary.

Movement!

Think that ultrasound was exciting? Just wait until you feel your little gymnast stretch and push inside of you for the first time.

So what does it feel like? It's often described in terms of butterfly wings or bubbles, or less poetically as gas or a block of jiggling Jello in the abdomen. Because pregnancy can cause so many gastrointestinal symptoms, you may not even notice the gentle nudges of baby until she's been persistent with her movements for a few days. You'll quickly discover that your baby is establishing behavioral patterns. When you're up and about, she may be rocked to sleep by your movements. It's when you lay down and try to take a rest that she wants to get up and groove. Have your partner stand by during a down time and see if he can catch a kick or two.

Once baby starts moving, the sensation becomes second nature. On average, you should feel four or more movements each hour. Three or fewer movements or a sudden decrease in fetal activity could be a sign of fetal distress, so if you notice either call your provider as soon as possible to follow up.

At the Doctor

If you didn't get to listen to the fetal heartbeat last month, you'll likely get your chance with this visit. Women who have chosen to take an alpha-fetoprotein (AFP) test will have their blood drawn sometime between weeks sixteen and eighteen.

Exercise

Don't avoid the gym, pool, or other favorite fitness hangouts just because you're pregnant. Exercise will not only make you feel better, it can tone muscles that will be getting a workout in labor and delivery. Feeling alarmingly large among the gym babes? Try mixing up your routine with something new like hiking, golf (sans cart), or a prenatal exercise class.

So how much is too much? It depends upon your prepregnancy fitness level. If you were swimming one hour each day before pregnancy, there's no reason not to continue that routine if you have your provider's blessing. On the other hand, don't start training for a marathon if your notion of exercise is walking into McDonald's instead of using the drive-thru. The rule of thumb—for women in "regular" pregnancies (i.e., not high-risk), thirty minutes of moderate exercise daily is ideal.

Precautions

While exercise can be a boon to your body and baby, there are basic steps you should take to stay safe.

·············· **need to know** ··············

First and foremost, run your routine by your provider to get a medical stamp of approval. If you're new to working out, start slowly.

Be attuned to your body's signals and stop immediately if you experience warning signs such as abdominal or chest pain, vaginal bleeding, dizziness, blurred vision, severe headache, or excessive shortness of breath. Dress in supportive, yet comfortable clothing. If your feet have swollen past the comfort level of your old gym shoes, invest in a bigger pair. Drink plenty of caffeine-free fluids before, during, and after your workout to remain well hydrated, and try to work out in a climate-controlled environment to avoid an extreme rise in core body temperature, as overheating can be hazardous to a developing fetus.

Kegels are one exercise every pregnant woman should know and practice. They strengthen the pelvic muscles for delivery and can improve the urinary incontinence, or dribbling, some women experience in pregnancy. What's a Kegel? Tighten the muscles you use to shut off your urine flow, hold for four seconds, and relax. You've just done your first Kegel. Try to work up to ten minutes of Kegels daily.

The Fifth Month

this month's priorities

○ Write down your symptoms.   ○ Track the fetal condition.

○ Monitor for diabetes.   ○ Plan for life after birth.

Baby This Month

At ten to twelve inches long and around one pound in weight, your baby is about the size of a regulation NFL football.

Your child is starting to bulk up a bit as she accumulates deposits of fat under her skin. A look at her through ultrasound might reveal a wave of her clenched hands. The fetus is now covered in a white oily substance known as vernix caseosa, a sort of full-body fetal Chapstick that keeps her fluid-soaked skin from peeling and protects against infection.

Your Body Changes

Feeling like you're turning inside out? Your "innie" may have already become an "outtie" as the skin of your belly is stretching, tightening, and itching like crazy. A good moisturizing cream can relieve the itching and keep your skin hydrated, although it won't prevent or eliminate striae gravidarum, or stretch marks.

> ·········· **need to know** ··························
>
> Whether or not you'll develop stretch marks is largely a matter of genetics, although factors such as excessive weight gain and multiple gestations may increase your odds of having them.

The red, purple, or whitish lines of striae are created by the excess collagen your body produces in response to rapid stretching of the skin. They may appear on your abdomen, breasts, or any other blossoming body part right now. Don't be too alarmed, as striae typically fade to virtually invisible silver lines after pregnancy.

What You Feel Like

The band of ligaments supporting your uterus is carrying an increasingly heavy load. You may start to feel occasional discomfort in your lower abdomen, inner thighs, and hips called round ligament pain. Pelvic tilt exercises are useful for keeping pelvic muscles toned and relieving pain. The pelvic tilt can be performed while standing against a wall but may be most comfortable done four-on-the-floor style.

The root of all things uncomfortable—pregnancy hormones—are also contributing to the lower back pain you may be experiencing. Progesterone and relaxin—the hormone responsible for softening your pelvic ligaments for delivery—are also loosening up your lower back ligaments and disks, and combined with the weight of your growing belly your back is feeling the strain. A few tips to help you ease your aches and pains:

Stand tall. Try to keep your center of gravity in your spine and pelvis rather than out in your belly, which can give you a swayback.

Sit up straight. Use good posture when you're sitting as well, and choose a chair with good lower back support

Avoid twists and turns. With everything so loose, a move as simple as quickly turning at the waist to get out of bed may strain your back. Use your arms as support for a slow take-off when rising from a chair.

continued

Practice your pickups. If you have small children that still need to be lifted occasionally, it's essential to use good form. To avoid injury, bend and use your leg muscles to lift things rather than bending from the waist and lifting with your back.

Warm up. A warm pad on your back, hips, or other sore spots may help relieve pain.

Foot rest. Use a low stool or step to rest your feet when sitting. If you must stand for long periods, alternate resting each foot on a step.

Massage. You now have a medical excuse to indulge in a regular back rub from your significant other. A licensed massage therapist who is experienced in prenatal massage may also be helpful.

Fluff and stuff. Sleep on your side with a pillow placed between your legs. This will align your spine and improve your sleeping posture.

Exercise. Check with your health care provider for approval and recommendations; if the pain is troublesome enough or if you have a history of back problems, she may suggest a physical therapist to work with.

At the Doctor

Beyond the usual weigh and measure routine, your doctor may administer a glucose tolerance test (GTT) at the end of the month (between weeks twenty-four and twenty-eight). If she hasn't discussed counting fetal movements before, she may mention it now.

.... **need to know** ....

Now that you're halfway through pregnancy, you may be thinking more about labor and delivery issues. It's never too early to ask your doctor questions about what's on your mind.

It's also a good time to start gathering information on childbirth classes from your local hospital or birthing center. There are several different methods of childbirth education, such as Lamaze, Bradley, and Bing; researching them now will give you and your partner time to learn more about which one is right for you. Register early, but try to pick a class date that falls in your third trimester so the information will still be fresh in your mind once the big day arrives.

Sleeping Tight

Perhaps it's nature's way of preparing you for the sleepless nights to come, but your growing belly and the pushes and prods of your little one are making it increasingly difficult to get the requisite eight or more hours of peaceful slumber. Sleep is essential to your mental and physical fitness right now, not to mention to that of your child. Make your best effort to rest often and rest well.

The fetal sleep cycle is only between twenty and eighty minutes long, so if you aren't a sound sleeper you may find yourself awakened by baby's stretching limbs. Logistically and medically, the best position for sleep right now is on your side.

················· **pregnancy treat** ·················

If you don't have one already, and it's in the budget, contemplate upgrading to a king-size bed. The extra room will enable you to bring a body pillow or beanbag into bed to support your stomach and ease your back.

Hip and shoulder pain may be another source of sleepless nights, and one that's difficult to avoid since you must sleep on your side. If you've tried the tips for aches and pains outlined above and the pain is still keeping you awake, experiment with a foam egg crate cushion on your mattress for a little added padding.

Your partner will also benefit from a bigger bed as he'll be less likely to waken at every toss and turn. Another bedroom habit you may have picked up in pregnancy is snoring. The snoring may be related to a number of factors, including pregnancy-related nasal congestion, your increased need for oxygen, swollen airway tissues, and compression of the muscles that control breathing. Your snoring will likely fade away after pregnancy. For now, invest in extra earplugs for your mate. Make sure your environment is as sleep-friendly as possible. The room temperature should be cool enough for your overheated metabolism; your partner may want to stock up on extra blankets to get him through these occasional chilly nights. If ambient noise is a problem, get some earplugs or a white noise conditioner to cut the clamor. More tips for preparing yourself for a good night's sleep:

- To avoid heartburn, don't eat immediately before bunking down, and have an extra pillow on hand to elevate your head.
- Make the bathroom the last stop before bed.
- Stock your nightstand with crackers if you wake with an unsettled stomach.
- If tender breasts are keeping you awake, wear a supportive bra to bed.
- Stay away from caffeine (it isn't the best thing for you right now anyway).
- Don't exercise up to three hours before bedtime.

The Sixth Month

this month's priorities

- ○ Bring up your fears with friends, family, experts, and other moms.
- ○ Browse in a baby store and start planning baby's room.
- ○ Make a list of must-have infant essentials and start stocking up on them.
- ○ Start thinking of names.

Baby This Month

Feeling a rhythmic lurch in your abdomen? Your little guy probably has the hiccups, a common phenomenon thought to be brought on by drinking and/or breathing amniotic fluid. They'll go away on their own, eventually; in the meantime, enjoy your little drummer boy and take advantage of the beat to let your partner feel the baby move.

The once-transparent skin of your fetus is starting to thicken, and sweat glands are developing below the skin surface. He's over a foot long now, and by the end of the month may weigh up to two pounds. He may now startle to a loud noise or other stimulation. Because his auditory system (has developed enough to sense and even discriminate among sounds readily, he is becoming accustomed to your voice and others who talk "to" him frequently.

need to know

Studies have demonstrated that newborns show a clear preference for their mother's voice, and for songs they heard while in the womb. Now is a good time to brush up on your lullaby repertoire.

Some clinical studies have found an association between exposure to excessive noise during pregnancy and high-frequency hearing loss in newborns. To stay on the safe side, you may want to avoid concerts, clubs, and other high-volume environments now. If your job involves heavy noise exposure, talk with your doctor about possible risks.

Your Body Changes

If the shoe fits . . . consider yourself lucky. What's behind all the swelling? The dramatic increase in blood volume you've experienced to nurture your child is feeding excess fluids to surrounding tissues, resulting in water retention. To make matters worse, the weight of your uterus is requiring the veins in your legs to work double time to pump all that extra blood back to the heart. And, of course, another culprit is pregnancy hormones, as estrogen increases the amount of fluid your tissues absorb. The result of all this is puffy and sometimes aching feet.

Special compression stockings, available at medical supply stores, may also be helpful. Don't restrict fluids or sodium—although avoiding excess sodium intake is fine, you actually need slightly more sodium in your diet in pregnancy to maintain your electrolyte balance. Fluids are crucial as well to prevent dehydration and keep you and baby well.

pregnancy treat

Putting your feet up when you can, wearing comfortable low-heeled shoes, and soaking your feet in cool water are all good ways to ease the discomfort.

What You Feel Like

You may have added leg cramps to your laundry list of pregnancy complaints. Stretching out your calf muscles can often quash a cramp, so the next time one hits extend your legs and point your toes toward your head.

A number of studies have found that oral magnesium supplementation can be useful in alleviating cramps in some women. Check with your health care provider to see what she suggests. Leg cramps can also be triggered by compression of your sciatic nerve—a condition commonly known as sciatica. Sciatica can also cause numbness and burning pain down the length of your leg and in your lower back and buttocks. Try stretching, a warm compress, or a tub soak for relief. If sciatica becomes more than a minor annoyance, talk to your health care provider.

At the Doctor

More of the same this month as your provider checks your weight and fundal height, listens to baby's heartbeat, and finds out about any new pregnancy symptoms you may be experiencing. If you're reporting swelling, your provider may check your feet and hands. And, of course, no prenatal visit is complete without a urine sample and blood pressure check. If you weren't given a glucose tolerance test to screen for gestational diabetes last month, it will probably be administered now.

Chapter 3

What Happened to My Ankles?: The Third Trimester

I t's the home stretch, the final act, the big countdown—the third trimester. You've made a lot of decisions so far, and there are even more to be made this month. Full speed ahead with labor and delivery preparations this month as you schedule childbirth classes and start to assemble a birth plan.

The Seventh Month

this month's priorities

○ If you haven't already signed up for childbirth classes, do so now.

○ Go over important issues with your doctor.

○ Schedule a tour of the hospital or birthing center where you plan to deliver.

○ Learn all the signs of premature labor.

Baby This Month

Weighing in at four pounds and about sixteen inches long, your baby is growing amazingly fast now. Her red, wrinkled skin is losing its fine lanugo covering as more insulating fat accumulates. And her eyelids, closed for so long, can now open and afford her a dim view of the place she will call home for just a few more months.

Dramatic developments in the brain and central nervous system are also occurring, as baby's nerve cells are sheathed with a substance called myelin that speeds nerve impulses. A seven-month-old fetus feels pain, can cry, and responds to stimulation from light or sound outside the womb. Her gymnastics may subside as her space gets smaller, but you're feeling her more intensely now and her movements may even be visible to both you and your partner. Even though your fetus is still producing lung surfactant and developing alveoli (air sacs), her lungs still aren't developed enough to breathe in the outside world.

Your Body Changes

The top of the fundus is halfway between your belly button and your breastbone, displacing your stomach, intestines, and diaphragm. Your expanding abdomen has formed a shelf. Not only are your breasts heavier, but they are also more glandular and getting ready to feed your baby. In this last trimester, your nipples may begin to leak colostrum, which is the yellowish, nutrient-rich fluid that precedes real breastmilk. To reduce backaches and breast tenderness, make sure you wear a well-fitting bra (even to bed if it helps). If you are planning on breastfeeding, you may want to consider buying some supportive nursing bras now that can take you through the rest of pregnancy and right into the postpartum period.

What You Feel Like

Your body is warming up for labor, and you may start to experience Braxton-Hicks contractions. These painless and irregular contractions feel as if your uterus is making a fist and then gradually relaxing it. If your little one is fairly active, you may think that she is stretching herself sideways at first. A quick check of your belly may reveal a visible tightening.

```
········· need to know ·········

Braxton-Hicks can begin as early as week twenty and continue right up
until your due date, although they're more commonly felt in the final month
of pregnancy.
```

Some first-time moms-to-be are afraid they won't be able to tell the difference between Braxton-Hicks and actual labor contractions. As any woman who has been through labor will attest, when the real thing comes you'll know it. Rule of thumb: if it hurts, it's labor.

Braxton-Hicks do not cause any changes to the cervix and occur at irregular intervals. They may even be uncomfortable at times but will usually subside if you change positions, another way to distinguish

Braxton-Hicks from the real thing. The actual definition of labor, even when it is premature, is the onset of regular, painful, uterine contractions that lead to a change in the cervix. If your contractions suddenly seem to be coming at regular intervals and they start to cause you pain or discomfort, they may be the real thing. Lie down on your left side for about a half-hour with a clock or watch on hand, and time the contractions from the beginning of one to the beginning of the next. If the interludes are more or less regular, call your health care provider. And if contractions of any type are accompanied by blood or amniotic fluid leakage, contact your practitioner immediately.

At the Doctor

Starting with this initial third-trimester visit, your visits to the doctor may start to step up to twice monthly. Your provider will probably want to know if you've been experiencing any Braxton-Hicks contractions, and he will cover the warning signs of preterm labor and what you should do if you experience them. If you're unsure about what type of childbirth class you'd like to take, you might want to bring your questions to your provider for her input. Just remember, the decision is ultimately up to you and your partner.

Women who are Rh negative will need treatment with Rh immune globulin (RhoGAM) this month. An injection is typically given at about twenty-eight weeks to protect the fetus from developing hemolytic disease—a condition in which the mother's antibodies attack the fetal red blood cells.

The Eighth Month

this month's priorities

○ Go to childbirth classes, and take your coach along.

○ Rethink your exercise routine.

○ Choose a pediatrician.

○ Prepare your hospital bag.

○ Prepare your baby's hospital bag.

Baby This Month

Gradually shifting to the same position in which 95 percent of all babies are born, your fetus starts to move into a head down pose, known as the vertex position. The small but stubborn percentage that don't assume the vertex position are considered breech. Feel a lot of kicking on your pelvic floor? It may be a clue that baby is still standing, or sitting, tall. She may also be lounging in the transverse position, or sideways in the womb.

Your little girl or boy is now up to 18 inches long and as heavy as a five-pound sack of flour. The rest of her body is finally catching up to the size of her head. Although it may feel like she's constantly up and about, she's actually sleeping 90 to 95 percent of the day, a figure that will drop only slightly when she is born. If your child were born today, she'd have an excellent chance of surviving and eventually thriving outside the womb. However, she'd still be considered preterm or premature, just as any birth before thirty-seven weeks of gestation.

Your Body Changes

Weight gain should start to slow down this month. If it doesn't, however, don't cut your calorie intake below 2,600 to try and stop it. You need the extra energy for both of you. As baby settles firmly on your bladder, bathroom stops step up once again. You may experience some stress incontinence, which is minor dribbling or leakage of urine when you sneeze, laugh, or make other sudden movements. This will clear up postpartum. In the meantime, keep doing your Kegels, don't hold it in, and wear a pantyliner.

What You Feel Like

Your Weeble-like physique has you off-balance and generally klutzy. Be careful—you wobble and you can fall down. And, of course, those pregnancy hormones have loosened up your joints and relaxed your muscles to make you a bit of a butterfingers. Pregnancy-related fluid retention can actually change the shape of your eyes and trigger minor vision changes. Also at work is estrogen, which causes your eyes to be drier than normal and may make contact lenses uncomfortable right now. It's easier and easier to get winded as your little one pushes up into your diaphragm. To ease breathing while you sleep, pile on a few extra pillows or use a foam bed wedge to elevate your head.

If you experience blurry vision or visual disturbances (e.g., spots) and you have high blood pressure or diabetes, let your provider know immediately. It could be a sign of poor control in both cases, which is dangerous to both you and your child.

At the Doctor

You'll see your provider twice this month as you continue your every-other-week routine. She will check the position of your baby to determine if he has turned head down in preparation for birth.

.... **need to know** ....

If your practitioner brings up the possibility of a breech (bottom or foot-first) birth, it's because she or he has felt the head of your unborn baby up near your ribs, or an ultrasound has confirmed that your child is in the breech position.

Your fickle fetus is likely to change position again in the next few weeks. If she doesn't, your practitioner may try to turn the baby closer to term using a technique known as external cephalic version, or manually attempting to turn the fetus in the uterus. The ACOG recommends that an external cephalic version be attempted in most breech cases. Babies can be delivered vaginally in breech position in some instances, but the procedure is more difficult and carries a higher risk for the infant. C-section is the method of choice for safe breech delivery. If you really want a vaginal birth and a cephalic version is unsuccessful in turning your breech, some practitioners may agree to a trial of labor to see if your contracting uterus helps to turn the child.

The Ninth Month

this month's priorities

○ Read up on delivery.

○ Get organized for the first days of new motherhood.

○ Learn the basics of infant care.

Baby This Month

Your child is packing on about ½ pound per week as he prepares to make his big exit. At delivery, the average U.S. birth weight is between 6 pounds, 10 ounces, to 7 pounds, 11 ounces.

He's fully formed and just waiting for the right time now. His lungs, the last organ system to fully mature, now have an adequate level of surfactant in them to allow breathing outside of the womb. A dark, tarry amalgam of amniotic fluid, skin cells, and other fetal waste, is gathering in your baby's intestines. This substance, called meconium, will become the contents of his bowel movements during the first few days of life.

Your Body Changes

Engagement or lightening, the process of the baby "dropping" down into the pelvic cavity in preparation for delivery, may occur any time now. In some women (particularly those who have given birth before), it may not happen until labor starts. Your cervix is softening in preparation for baby's passage. As it effaces (thins) and dilates (opens), the soft plug of mucus keeping it sealed tight may be dislodged. This mass, which the appealing name of mucus plug, may be tinged red or pink and is also referred to as the equally explicit bloody show.

What You Feel Like

If the baby has dropped, you may be running to the bathroom more than ever. He also may be sending shockwaves through your pelvis as he settles further down onto the pelvic floor. On the upside, you can finally breathe as he pulls away from your lungs and diaphragm. Braxton-Hicks contractions may be more frequent this month as you draw nearer to delivery. You're close enough to be on the lookout for the real thing, however. How will you recognize them? Real contractions will:

- Be felt in the back and possibly radiate around to the abdomen.
- Not subside when you move around or change positions.
- Increase in intensity as time passes and come at roughly regular intervals (early on this may be from twenty to forty-five minutes apart).
- Increase in intensity with activity like walking.

Other signs that labor is on its way include amniotic fluid leaks in either a gush or a trickle (your "water breaking"), sudden diarrhea, and the appearance of the mucus plug. Keep in mind, however, that for many women, the bag of waters does not break until active labor sets in.

At the Doctor

You'll see your doctor on a weekly basis now until you deliver. Unless you are scheduled for a planned caesarean, your provider will probably perform an internal exam with each visit to check your cervix for changes that indicate approaching labor.

••••••••••••••••••••• **need to know** •••••••••••••••••••••

The U.S. Center for Disease Control recommends that your provider administer a group B strep (GBS) test one month prior to your estimated delivery date. This culture is performed by swabbing a fluid sample from both your vagina and rectum. If the cultured fluid comes back positive for GBS, you may have antibiotics administered during delivery to prevent transmission to the baby.

Your provider will be checking your cervix for signs that it is preparing for your baby's passage. She'll also be taking note of any descent or dropping of the baby toward the pelvis, called the station. Although you may start effacing and dilating now, it's still anyone's guess as to when labor will begin, and it could be a few more weeks yet.

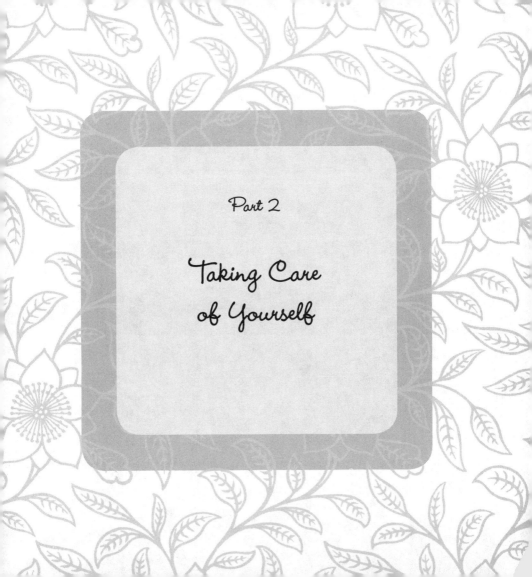

Part 2

Taking Care
of Yourself

Chapter 4

Who Should Be Present at the Birth— and Where to Have Your Baby

irth is perhaps the most profound event you'll experience in your lifetime. It involves not just a transformation of your body and the launch of a new life but an evolution of the self. Preparing your body and clearing your mind of any anxieties and preconceptions about the birth process are the best ways to get ready for a wonderful birth experience.

Selecting Birth Partners

Who will help guide you in your birth journey? It's an important decision that you shouldn't leave up to the Yellow Pages. Ask yourself where your comfort zone lies.

Does having an obstetrician in attendance give you additional peace of mind? Do you feel more at ease with an experienced midwife and doula on your team? Or is an intimate birth experience with one-on-one midwife care more your style?

Your Team

Choosing the people that will attend your birth is one of the most important and far-reaching decisions you'll make about your birth experience. Having a clinically competent and empathetic team in your corner can make even the most difficult birth a positive experience.

······················· **need to know** ·······················

Consider the three essential Cs—communication, comfort, and connection. Your birth partner needs to be someone you can talk to openly and frankly and who won't be afraid to be candid with you as well.

Check with your health insurer before selecting your care providers for your birth. Some insurers may have restrictions on coverage for midwives who are not certified nurse-midwives (CNMs). They may also limit coverage on doula services. Many midwives and doulas will offer sliding scale fees to offset costs if coverage is a problem. If you already see a gynecologist or family-practice doctor with an obstetric practice and have forged a good patient-doctor relationship with him or her, your search may be already over. If you're looking for a new provider, your options include these:

A midwife. Midwives may be either certified nurse-midwives (CNMs), direct entry midwives (DEMs), or licensed midwives (LMs). Their focus is on patient-directed care in pregnancy, labor, and delivery.

An ob/gyn. An obstetrician and gynecologist is an M.D. who has completed training in women's health and reproductive medicine.

A doula. Unlike a midwife or ob/gyn, a doula's sole purpose is for emotional support during delivery.

Many of today's obstetrical practices are combined, employing midwives, nurse-practitioners, and ob/gyns. Sometimes you will have a choice of seeing one or more different types of providers throughout your pregnancy.

It's never too late to change health-care providers. If you've been seeing someone for prenatal care and have found that you have irreconcilable philosophical differences about your impending birth, do not hesitate to start looking for someone you can work with. Other mothers are great sources of information on midwives, obstetricians, and doulas.

Choosing Wisely

Remember that some of your wishes for your baby's birth may already narrow down the playing field for choosing a practitioner. For example, if you want a home birth, you will probably be choosing a midwife, since virtually no physicians will attend a home birth because of liability issues.

Don't be afraid to interview your potential candidates before committing to a decision. Following are some things to ask your interviewees.

Who will deliver my baby? Will the doctor or midwife you choose deliver your child, or is there a possibility it will be another provider within their practice? Who provides backup care for them during downtime and emergencies, and will you have the opportunity to meet that person before the birth?

What hospital or birthing center are you affiliated with? Where your birth will take place will be an important part of the birth experience.

Do you encourage birth plans? Will the provider honor your wishes as outlined in a birth plan and work with you to explore options should things veer off course? Will the plan be submitted into your chart so those in attendance at your birth will have access to it?

What is your philosophy on pain relief and birth interventions? If you have strong feelings about pain-relief choices and interventions like episiotomy, here's your chance to find out if your provider will work with you toward the birth you want.

How can I reach you in an emergency? Find out the triage procedure for calls to the office and whether the provider is available by pager or cell phone.

Making sure your birthing practitioner understands what is important to you is an essential part of the birthing process, along with choosing where to have your baby.

Choosing the Birth Place That's Right for You

First and foremost, you want to be at ease in the place you choose to labor and give birth. Studies have shown that high anxiety levels in laboring women result in increased pain perception. The stress hormone cortisol can also delay lactation and lengthen labor.

Comfort is of course, subjective—some women feel reassured by a hospital setting, knowing that care for any potential medical problems is nearby. Others feel tense in such sterile surroundings and prefer the warmth of a birthing center or their own homes.

Considering Rules and Policies

In addition to personal perceptions of your environment, you also need to choose a place your provider can and will work in. You may have an ob/gyn you really like and trust, but if you want this person to deliver your baby, chances are you won't be able to have a home birth. And depending on state and hospital regulations where you live, a midwife may not be able to be the sole health-care professional overseeing your birth at the hospital. As a starting point, ask your provider about where he or she has privileges to work. You may end up deciding that the person is more important than the place, or vice versa.

According to the U.S. Center for Disease Control's National Center for Health Statistics (NCHS), of the more than 4 million births in the United States in 2001, 99 percent took place in a hospital setting. Of all out-of-hospital births in 2001, 28 percent took place in a freestanding birthing center, and 65 percent took place at home.

There are also facility rules and regulations to deal with when you choose a birth place. If you have certain expectations regarding how you will be allowed to labor and manage your pain, and they go against hospital guidelines, it could be a deal-breaker for you. On the other hand, some hospitals and birthing centers may be more flexible on these issues than others, so don't assume out of hand that your needs won't be met—ask questions first.

Birth in a Hospital

Today, many hospitals have introduced more family-friendly labor-delivery-recovery (LDR) rooms so women are able to spend their birth experience—labor, birth, and mother-baby bonding time—in the same room.

Again, your experience may vary, and your access to hospital amenities may be limited by your health plan and by where you live. If you think you want a hospital birth, call around and learn more about specific facilities and policies. Ask other women about their experiences delivering, and call up the patient advocate at each facility to ask more questions about what's expected of and offered to maternity patients. Take the time to investigate your options fully before the big day.

What's a patient advocate?

As the name implies, a patient advocate is an individual at the hospital charged with representing patient interests and bringing patient concerns to hospital administrators. They act as liaisons between the patients and the hospital staff. Not all hospitals employ patient advocates, but if the one you're considering does, these representatives can be a valuable resource for answering your questions.

Labor-Delivery-Recovery Room

The advent of the LDR room on hospital maternity wards has brought many of the appealing characteristics of a birthing center into the hospital. An LDR room has a warm and inviting atmosphere that resembles a bedroom more than a hospital room. Showers, whirlpool tubs, and other nontraditional pain relief amenities, as well as soft lighting and music, are just a few of the perks you might find in today's LDR rooms.

Some facilities have taken the "one-stop" approach even further, offering women LDRP rooms in which they can also spend their postpartum stay.

·············· pregnancy treat ··············

LDRP rooms may feature a pullout bed or other place for the new dad to bunk down, plus comfortable furniture for visiting family and friends. Some even offer special meal catering to the new parents as an alternative to typical hospital-cafeteria fare.

For those hospitals with LDR rooms, the mother is typically moved into a postpartum room for the duration of her hospital stay. How long that is depends on medical condition, physician assessment, insurance coverage, and state regulations, but in a typical uncomplicated birth, an inpatient stay usually won't exceed forty-eight to seventy-two hours. Under the federal Health Insurance Portability and Accountability Act (HIPPA), health insurers who offer maternity coverage cannot restrict coverage to less than forty-eight hours in a vaginal birth, or ninety-six hours in a C-section birth.

Rooming In

Another thing most hospitals have changed their ways about is keeping the new baby nursery-bound. Barring any neonatal complications, most new mothers are encouraged to have their infant "room-in" with them, going to the nursery only for checkups, weigh-ins, or when requested by mom. In addition to giving new mothers the opportunity to practice new baby care, rooming in promotes breastfeeding and mother-baby bonding.

If you choose a hospital birth, take advantage of your time as an inpatient to rest and replenish your strength after birth. Rooming-in is wonderful, but if you need some uninterrupted sleep (something you won't be getting much of after you return home), the nursery is there for your baby. ʳ be sure to let the nursing staff know your feeding preferences so they ˙ke you to breastfeed baby if necessary.

A Birthing-Center Birth Experience

In addition to their "almost-home" atmosphere, studies have found that birth centers have lower C-section rates and higher reported maternal satisfaction than their hospital counterparts. According to The National Birth Center Study, an analysis of more than 11,800 births taking place in eighty-four freestanding birth centers nationwide, the cesarean section rate for women receiving care in birth centers was approximately half that of women in low-risk, in-hospital births.

According to the National Association of Childbearing Centers (NACC), thirty-seven states currently license freestanding birthing centers. Some states require accreditation to grant licensure. Birth centers are accredited by the Commission for the Accreditation of Birth Centers (CABC), the accrediting arm of the NACC, and must meet certain quality-of-care, facility, and personnel guidelines as outlined by the CABC.

Why Choose a Birthing Center?

Birthing centers are usually primarily midwife- and nurse-midwife–staffed and as such maintain a noninterventional philosophy toward birth. Things like continuous fetal monitoring, epidurals, and surgical interventions (including C-section or episiotomy) are not routinely practiced. As such, many centers will only take low-risk, uncomplicated births. Physicians are often on staff on a consultant basis should the need arise for specialized medical advice or care. Because complications can occur during even a low-risk birth, birthing centers have a transport protocol in place to move women who develop labor complications to a nearby hospital.

••••••••••••••••••• **need to know** •••••••••••••••••••

Many birthing centers also offer onsite prenatal and postpartum care, allowing you to develop a relationship with your midwife and become familiar with the center facilities well before the birth itself.

Some of the other benefits of birthing centers include the following:

Freedom. Women can labor in whatever position they want, not tethered to a monitor or IV line.

Peace. A birth center is typically a quiet place, something not true of most hospitals.

Solitude. While a maternity ward in an urban hospital may have up to several dozen women laboring at once, the birth center typically has one or two births simultaneously.

Brevity. Most women are discharged between four and nine hours postpartum, versus the forty-eight- to seventy-two-hour hospital stay for inpatient births.

the "i have a life" pregnancy guide

Continuity. In most cases, the same midwife will stay with a woman throughout the birth instead of leaving with shift changes.

Cost-efficiency. In addition to the cost saving from a shorter stay, birthing-center births save money by minimizing costly technological interventions.

Strength. Birthing centers tend to focus on preventative care and instilling a sense of self-sufficiency and self-awareness in women regarding their own health and abilities.

Balance. For many women, the birth center offers a good middle ground between hospital and home.

When interviewing birth centers, be sure to ask what their transfer protocol is should complications arise, and what sort of complications would mandate a transfer to a hospital. You may or may not be able to stay under the care of your midwife if a transfer occurs, so be sure to inquire if she will continue your care at the hospital.

Home Birth

What better place to welcome your child into the world than the cradle of your family—your home? This is the one place where you can completely relax, be yourself, and labor in any way, shape, or form.

Home birth offers all the comforts and many of the perks of the birthing center. And for women who don't want a hospital birth, but may be excluded by a birthing center's "low-risk" selection protocols because they are having twins or because they have had a previous C-section, an attended home birth may provide them the birth experience they want. However, home birth is not without risks. A woman who is already in a "high-risk" situation should have a careful discussion with her health-care provider to go over the options available based on her particular situation and health history.

····················· **need to know** ·····················

> The American Medical Association (AMA) and the American College of Obstetricians and Gynecologists (ACOG) are squarely against home births, citing safety as a concern.

If you choose home birth, talk to your midwife about the supplies you should have on hand. Home birth "kits"—which include such essential items as plastic sheeting, cotton balls, and compresses—are available for purchase from childbirth retailers. You can also assemble the components from a list your midwife provides. Finally, if you don't have a big bathtub but would love to labor in a Jacuzzi, rental birthing-tubs are an option. Your midwife or doula can provide more information.

If you live in a rural or isolated area and an emergency situation arises, you won't have the benefits of immediate medical care that a hospital can provide. A good midwife who carries resuscitation equipment and has a transport plan and protocol in place can help minimize some of the risks related to complications.

In response, home-birth advocates point to research that backs up both the safety and effectiveness of the home setting for planned term low-risk births.

What to Ask

The best way to avoid any stressful misunderstandings during the birth itself is to clarify all the rules and regulations well in advance. Talk to the hospital or birthing center staff (or in the case of home birth, your provider), and find out what the guidelines are.

If you're planning a birthing center or hospital birth and will also be attending childbirth preparation classes at the same facility, you'll have an opportunity to ask questions in class. Many centers or hospitals will provide printed information in class that details facility guidelines and may answer many of your questions for you. In addition, facility tours are usually an integral part of childbirth preparation classes.

One advantage of many birthing centers is that you have plenty of opportunities for follow-up questions during routine prenatal care visits, since your provider will typically take appointments at the center. But wherever you plan your birth, don't hesitate to pick up the phone and call the facility with any concerns or questions.

For the Hospital and Birthing Center

If you are planning to check in to a hospital or birthing center, it's important that you know what to expect. If you have any specific personal requirements, asking questions early will help you find a facility that will accommodate you. Here are some questions to ask:

- Can I wear my own clothes to labor in?
- What is your fetal monitoring policy?
- Can I eat and/or drink at will during labor?
- Are there limitations on whom I have present during the birth?
- Can I walk and choose my own positions to labor in?
- If I want pharmaceutical pain relief, what are my options?
- Are there any mandatory interventions, such as an intravenous line?
- Can my partner film the birth?
- May I labor in a tub or shower?
- May I give birth in the tub/underwater should I choose to do so?
- What is your emergency transport procedure?
- Do you accept and honor birth plans?
- What is the cesarean rate of the hospital? (Note: It's also important to find out what your provider's individual C-section rate is.)
- Is the birth center licensed by the state? Is it accredited by the National Association for Childbearing Centers (NACC)?
- Will I be consulted about and be the primary decision maker regarding birth interventions?

Questions for Home–Birth Care Providers

Most home births are performed by midwives. Although some physicians will attend a home birth, liability and malpractice issues prevent many from doing so. Some questions to ask your provider if you're considering home birth are the following:

- How early in labor will you arrive for the birth?
- What emergency and resuscitation equipment do you have available?
- If complications occur, what is your procedure for handling them?
- Do I need to assemble home birth supplies or are they supplied by you and included in your fee?
- How many births have you attended?
- What pain relief techniques do you use?
- If I want pharmaceutical pain relief, what are my options?
- Do you place a limit on the support people present during the birth itself?
- What is your episiotomy rate?
- What tasks will you perform after the birth in terms of cleanup?
- What is your procedure for examining and disposing of the placenta?

Provider and Insurance Issues

It probably goes without saying that you should check your insurance coverage for participating providers and facilities when deciding on your birth place. If you'd like to have a home birth, there's a good chance it may not be covered by your health-insurance provider. That doesn't mean that you automatically need to take no for an answer. First of all, leave a paper trail. Remember that any assurances or denials you get on coverage should be in black and white. If you don't see home-birth coverage in your policy, but during a phone consultation an insurance representative assures you that you're covered, ask for written confirmation of coverage to be mailed to you on company letterhead. The same goes for a denial of coverage.

If your insurer does deny home-birth coverage, call your state department of insurance or business regulation and ask what the regulatory guidelines are regarding midwife and home-birth coverage and insurance restrictions so you know your rights. Again, ask for a hard copy of the specific legislation, or at least get a citation so you can look it up for yourself.

·········· **need to know** ··········

Find out what the appeals process is for your health insurer and file a written appeal. It may help to include citations of published clinical studies that have demonstrated the safety and cost-savings of home birth.

Your midwife or health-care provider should be able to help you with specific references. Send a copy of your appeal to the state regulatory agency.

If your insurer still denies your claim, find out the process for filing a complaint with your state insurance regulatory body, and do so. Make sure you send your insurer a copy. Finally, if your health insurance plan is through your employer, talk to your human resources contact about the issue. He or she may be able to assist you in your appeal. At the least, if your human resources department is aware of the denial and you make them aware of the financial and medical benefits of home birth, they may reconsider doing business with the insurer when it's time to renew plan contracts.

If you do end up paying out of pocket, talk to your midwife well in advance of your due date to discuss your payment options. An installment agreement or sliding scale fees (if your provider offers them) may make the cost more affordable.

Chapter 5

What Are All Those Tests For?

*Y*ou'll be poked, prodded, swabbed, scraped, and scanned throughout your pregnancy. All these tests have a purpose, of course—a healthy mom and baby. This chapter gives you a rundown of what you have to look forward to and what it all means.

Urine Tests

You'll be giving a urine sample at each prenatal visit for urinalysis. Your provider's office or lab will test your urine for ketones, protein, and glucose at each visit and may also check for the presence of any bacteria.

Ketones

Ketone bodies are substances produced when the body is getting insufficient fuel from food intake and has to metabolize fat for energy. The result is a process known as ketosis, and the resulting ketones spill into the urine. Ketones may appear in pregnancy if you're suffering from severe nausea and vomiting, and they are a sign that you may require intravenous nutrition. They can also be a byproduct of gestational diabetes when blood sugars get too high (above 200 mg/dl) and can lead to a potential life-threatening complication called diabetic ketoacidosis (DKA). The ketone test is generally performed with a reagent test strip, where a strip of chemically treated paper is dipped in your urine sample and then matched against a color chart for the presence of ketones. Test strips allow your provider or her staff to get fairly instantaneous results.

Protein

Excessive protein (albumin) in the urine can be a sign of preeclampsia (also known as toxemia or pregnancy induced hypertension). It is also a possible indication of urinary tract infection (UTI) or renal (kidney) impairment. The presence of white blood cells in urine can be an indication of infection as well. Your provider will again use a test strip to check for protein.

If the strip is positive, it indicates that protein levels above 30 mg/dl are detected, which is considered more than the trace amount normally present in urine. A positive protein strip is an indication for further testing with the more specific twenty-four-hour urine test. In a twenty-four-hour urine test, you'll be given a special container to collect your urine in, and you'll be asked to keep the sample refrigerated during the collection period. Pregnant women typically excrete 260 milligrams of protein or less in a twenty-four-hour period. If preeclampsia is suspected, your provider will probably order additional tests.

Glucose

Glucose, or sugar, in the urine (called glycosuria) may be a sign of gestational diabetes mellitus (GDM). It's normal to spill a small amount of sugar into the urine in pregnancy, but consistent high levels along with other risk factors raise a red flag that GDM may be present. Again, test reagent strips are used for screening. If your doctor suspects GDM, she will order a glucose challenge test (GCT). If this is abnormal, she'll then order an oral glucose tolerance test (GTT; see "Blood Work" following).

Urine Culture

Your urine will be analyzed and cultured for the presence of bacteria at your first prenatal visit, and again during pregnancy if symptoms of a urinary tract infection (e.g., burning during urination, strong smelling urine) appear.

Blood Work

You won't be handing out your blood as frequently as your urine, but there still are a few blood tests involved in pregnancy.

Hemoglobin Count

Your hemoglobin levels, the red blood cells that carry oxygen throughout your body, will be assessed at your initial prenatal visit and may be tested again in the second and third trimesters. Low hemoglobin levels, called anemia, occur frequently in pregnancy due to the vast boost of your total blood volume product. Levels that are too low can be a risk factor for low birth weight babies. If your total hemoglobin levels are below 12 mg/dl, your provider may prescribe iron supplements to build your hemoglobin reserves and order regular hemoglobin screenings at each prenatal visit to monitor your progress.

Glucose Challenge

The glucose challenge test is a screening tool for gestational diabetes mellitus (GDM). It's typically given between twenty-four and twenty-eight weeks of pregnancy but may be administered earlier in women considered at risk for GDM. You may be instructed to carbo load before the test, and then will be given 50 grams of a glucose solution, usually what is known as Glucola, to drink. One hour later, blood will be drawn and your blood serum glucose levels will be measured. A level greater than 135–140 mg/dl is considered high, in which case further testing will be necessary.

Oral Glucose Tolerance Test (GTT)

Women who test with high serum glucose levels after the glucose challenge are then given an oral glucose tolerance test to make a definitive diagnosis of gestational diabetes. The GTT, or three-hour glucose challenge, is a fasting test. Since pregnancy and fasting don't mix too well, the test is typically administered first thing in the morning. When you arrive at the lab, blood will be taken, then you will be given 100 grams of Glucola to drink. Your blood will be drawn at one-hour intervals until you reach the three-hour mark. The glucose levels in the blood samples you provide will be analyzed and checked against the diagnostic criteria for GDM. The American Diabetes Association recommends lab values known as the Carpenter and Coustan scale for interpreting GTT results. A level of 95 mg/dl or higher at the start of the test, 180 mg/dl or higher at one hour, 155 mg/dl or higher at two hours, and 140 mg/dl or higher at three hours is considered elevated. If two or more levels are elevated, a diagnosis of gestational diabetes is given.

Other Blood Tests

Your blood type and rhesus, or Rh, factor will be determined at your first prenatal visit. An Rh factor is either positive or negative. If your Rh is positive, no treatment is necessary. If you are Rh negative, you are at risk for Rh incompatibility with the blood type of your baby. Rh incompatibility occurs when your unborn baby is Rh positive and your Rh negative blood combines with hers. When this happens, your immune system may try to fight off the baby as an intruder, causing serious complications. Receiving RhoGAM will prevent this from happening.

•••••••••••••••••••••••••••• need to know ••••••••••••••••••••••••

Blood tests also determine whether or not you are immune to German measles (rubella). German measles can cause birth defects, especially if you contract the infection during the first trimester, and can cause cataracts, heart defects, and deafness in offspring.

A majority of women have been exposed to the rubella virus or have been vaccinated against it before becoming pregnant, however, and immunity lasts a lifetime.

The ACOG now recommends that all pregnant couples, regardless of ethnic background, be offered cystic fibrosis screening. Blood tests can also screen for inherited anemia in at-risk populations. For example, couples of African, Caribbean, Eastern Mediterranean, Middle Eastern, and Asian descent are at risk for sickle cell anemia. Families of Greek, Italian, Turkish, African, West Indian, Arabian, or Asian descent may be screened for the thalassemia trait; if both father and mother are carriers, there is a chance that the fetus could develop the blood disease thalassemia major. The alpha-fetoprotein (AFP) blood tests, or variations called the triple or quad AFP screens, are used in pregnancy to screen for genetic problems and certain birth defects. If initial blood screening tests for genetic conditions are positive, an amniocentesis or CVS can help determine if the trait has been passed on to the baby. A trip to a genetic counselor to weigh all your options and assess their risks and benefits is a good idea.

Swabs and Smears

More bodily fluid tests will be taken throughout pregnancy, particularly at the initial prenatal workup. If you have not received a Pap smear in the last year, your doctor will give you one, which you are likely familiar with from gynecologist appointments. You will also have swabs or smears to test for other diseases or infections.

Group B Strep

Group B streptococcus (GBS) is a bacterium that can cause serious infections in a newborn—including pneumonia and meningitis. If a pregnant woman tests positive for it, she is usually prescribed intravenous antibiotics during labor and delivery to prevent transmission to her baby. Swabs of both the rectum and vagina are taken and cultured (put in a medium that will allow the bacteria to grow if it is present). The U.S. Center for Disease Control (CDC) advises that all pregnant women be screened for GBS at thirty-five to thirty-seven weeks gestation.

Sexually Transmitted Diseases (STDs)

The CDC also recommends that all pregnant women be screened for several sexually transmitted diseases because of their potentially devastating effects on a fetus. HIV, hepatitis B, and syphilis testing require a blood draw, while chlamydia and gonorrhea are tested with a polymerase chain reaction (PCR) test. You may only be offered some of these tests by your provider based on your medical history and perceived risk factors. If you'd like to be tested for all of them, ask your doctor.

Chlamydia, gonorrhea, and syphilis are caused by bacteria and can be treated with antibiotics. Viral infections like hepatitis B and HIV cannot be cured in the mother, but precautionary measures can greatly decrease the risks of her passing on the disease to her child during labor and delivery.

Ultrasounds

In addition to giving you your first glimpse at your little one, an ultrasound lets your practitioner assess the baby's growth and development. It may also be used to diagnose placental abnormalities, an ectopic pregnancy, certain birth defects, or other suspected problems.

.... **need to know** ....

There are two types of ultrasound scans: the transabdominal, which scans through your abdomen, and the transvaginal, which scans directly into your vagina.

In very early pregnancy, the technician may opt for the vaginal approach, which means that the transducer will be inserted into your vagina. However, abdominal ultrasounds are the most common as most ultrasounds take place in the second and the third trimesters. An ultrasound typically takes no longer than a half-hour to perform. If you are in the first half of your pregnancy, you will probably be instructed to drink plenty of water prior to the exam, and refrain from emptying your bladder. The extra fluids help the technician to visualize your baby. Once in the examining room, you will recline on a table or bed with your upper body elevated and your abdomen exposed. Ask for extra pillows if you tend to get woozy when not lying on your side. The lights may be dimmed to allow the operator to see the sonogram picture more clearly. A thin application of transducer paste, jelly, or oil will be spread on your abdomen and then the fun begins.

The ultrasound picture, or sonogram, is obtained when high-frequency sound waves are passed over your abdomen with a hand-held wand called a transducer. These waves bounce off the solid structures of your baby, sending back a moving image of the tiny being inside. The resulting picture is transmitted to a computer or television screen. Ultrasound pictures are typically a grainy black and white.

···················· **pregnancy treat** ····························

The ultrasound operator can print out pictures for you to take home, so if she doesn't offer, make sure you ask.

The ultrasound technician may take a series of measurements during the procedure with the computer attached to the machine. These measurements help your provider assess the growth and organ development of the fetus. Depending on the timing of the test and the cooperation of your unborn child, she may also be able to get an idea of his or her gender. Typically, this information won't be given unless you ask for it, in case you prefer to be surprised at birth.

When and if you have an ultrasound will depend upon your provider. Many obstetricians order ultrasounds as a matter of routine. Some do one at the first visit to check for correct dates and viability with the rationale that it may save them from questioning gestational dates later on (as dating is more accurate in the first trimester). Others will recommend a sonogram at around twenty weeks to examine the fetal anatomy and ensure the pregnancy is progressing normally. A patient's peace of mind may also be reason enough to order an ultrasound. Since it is a noninvasive and fairly inexpensive test that can reassure the parents that things are developing normally, many providers will comply with a woman's request for an ultrasound. If your doctor hasn't ordered one and you have some anxieties about your baby's health, it can't hurt to ask.

Alpha-fetoprotein (AFP)/ Triple or Quad Screen Test

Alpha-fetoprotein is a blood protein produced by your unborn baby and passed into your circulatory system. The AFP, administered between weeks sixteen and eighteen, is a blood test used to screen for chromosomal irregularities like trisomy 18 and Down syndrome, and also for neural tube defects. Results of this test are usually available in about a week.

Most of the time, a high level of AFP can be explained by multiple gestation (twins, triplets, or more). However, it could also mean that your fetus has a neural tube defect. If AFP levels are low, it may be an indication of Down syndrome, trisomy 18, or other chromosomal disorders. It could also mean that your dates are wrong. A level-one or level-two ultrasound or an amniocentesis may be ordered for further evaluation. You may also be referred to a genetic counselor. A more extensive version of the AFP, called the triple-screen test (or AFP-3), measures levels of human chorionic gonadotropin (hCG) and estriol, a type of estrogen, as well as AFP. The quad-test, an even more sensitive marker of chromosomal problems, assesses all three of these substances plus inhibin-A. A misdated pregnancy can affect the results of your AFP or triple or quad screen and give a false positive. An ultrasound can help to confirm or adjust the gestational age.

Amniocentesis

The thought of an amniocentesis makes many women nervous, probably because it involves two critical undertakings: a needle being inserted through the abdomen and breaching your baby's watery environment. It does carry some risk of complications, including a slight chance of miscarriage. However, the amnio (as it is commonly referred to) is one of the best tools available for diagnosing chromosomal abnormalities, genetic disorders, and birth defects.

.... **need to know** ....

An amniocentesis is typically performed in the second trimester after week 15 or 16 of pregnancy, although a later amnio may be done depending on the reason.

Your provider may suggest you meet with a genetic counselor prior to having an amniocentesis performed to weigh the risks versus the benefits of the procedure, given your specific medical background and family history. She will also lay out any alternative procedures that may be options, such as a level-two ultrasound. If you do decide to go with the amnio, you may be sent to a perinatologist, or maternal-fetal specialist, who is experienced in the procedure. An amniocentesis is a relatively short outpatient procedure. Your abdomen is first swabbed with an antiseptic solution. The physician will use the abdominal ultrasound procedure to see her way around your womb. She will then insert a needle into the amniotic sac and draw an amniotic fluid sample into a syringe. The fluid contains sloughed-off fetal cells, which will be analyzed in the lab. Here are reasons why an amniocentesis may be planned:

Age: Women over thirty-five have an increased risk of carrying a baby with a chromosomal disorder like Down syndrome. When the father is over fifty, amniocentesis could also be advised because there may be a connection between paternal age and an increased risk of Down syndrome.

Family history: If you've already had a baby with a hereditary or chromosomal abnormality or neural tube defects, an amniocentesis could make you feel more comfortable.

continued

Rh status: Rh negative women may have an amnio to determine the Rh status of their fetus.

AFP, triple screen, or quad-test results: If alpha-fetoprotein (AFP) shows up at a higher than normal level, an amnio may help clear up any questions.

Ultrasound abnormalities: If your ultrasound turned up indications of the possibility of a chromosomal disorder, an amnio may be recommended for further evaluation.

Lung maturity: If you're experiencing symptoms of preterm labor or other medical complications that point to an early birth, your provider may perform an amnio to check the level of surfactant present in the fluid, a marker of fetal lung maturity.

Infection: If you have preterm labor and your doctor is worried about an infection, an amnio may be recommended.

After the amnio procedure, the baby will be monitored by ultrasound and will have his heart rate checked for a few minutes to ensure that everything is okay. You may experience minimal cramping. You will be advised to restrict strenuous exercise for one day, although other normal activity should be fine. If in the days following amnio you experience fluid or blood discharge from the vagina, let your provider know as soon as possible.

There is also a slight risk of trauma to the unborn baby from a misplaced needle or inadvertent rupture of the sac. If there are problems, the information you get from an amnio can prepare you for providing your child with the best care possible at birth. However, the timing can make other decisions difficult. Results from your amniocentesis won't be available for up to two weeks. And by the time the test results are back, you will be halfway through your pregnancy (about twenty weeks). For this reason, some women at risk for chromosomal abnormalities will choose the chorionic villus sampling test, which can be performed in the first trimester, instead. A consultation with a genetic counselor can help you analyze the positives and negatives and decide if a CVS is right for you.

·············· **need to know** ··············

The U.S. Center for Disease Control and Prevention (CDC) estimates the chance of miscarriage following an amnio at somewhere between one in 400 and one in 200, and the risk of uterine infection at less than one in 1,000.

Fetal Monitoring

A fetal heart monitor measures—you guessed it—the fetal heart rate (or FHR). A baseline, or average, fetal heart rate of 120 to 160 beats per minute (bpm) is considered normal. Spikes as high as 25 bpm are normal and coincide with fetal stimulation and sleep cycles.

During Labor

Fetal monitors also measure the length and severity of contractions. There are both external and internal monitors available. An external monitor uses two belts that are positioned around your belly. The transducers on each are adjusted until they are both measuring your contractions and picking up the fetal heart sounds. If you are in a high-risk pregnancy, you may be hooked up to an internal fetal monitor during labor and delivery.

> ················ **need to know** ························
>
> Internal monitors may only be used in labor when the amniotic sac has broken. This monitor is considered more sensitive and accurate but is also more invasive.

It uses a little springlike wire that is inserted vaginally and sits just under the skin on the baby's head. Both internal and external monitoring can keep you tethered to your bed during labor, which may not be the experience you want. External monitors, however, can be removed for a short time, but in general fetal movement should be assessed at least every fifteen minutes.

Stress and Non-Stress Test (NST)

If there is any concern about fetal well-being or if you are still waiting for baby's belated arrival at forty-one or forty-two weeks, you'll probably be given a non-stress test. A non-stress test (NST) measures fetal heart rate and is performed any time after twenty-four weeks. When you move, your heart rate speeds up, and when baby moves, his heart rate speeds up, the sign of a healthy fetus. The test is administered on a bed or examining table attached to a fetal monitor. The monitor belts are strapped around your abdomen. For about twenty minutes, every time you feel your baby move, you'll push a button. The button will record the movement on the paper strip or computer record of baby's heartbeat. Depending on how the monitor is hooked up, it may also detect and note the movement. Rises in the FHR should correspond to fetal movement. If there is no movement, it's quite possible that baby is sleeping. You'll be given a drink of juice or small snack in an attempt to rouse her. Sometimes, a buzzer or vibrations called vibroacoustic stimulation are used to wake up a sleeping fetus. If these methods are unsuccessful, further testing is needed, and a biophysical profile (BPP) may be ordered. Fifteen percent of NSTs before thirty-two weeks are nonreactive. In a stress test (also called a contraction stress test or oxytocin challenge test), mild contractions are induced with the hormone Pitocin to see how your baby responds. You will be hooked up to a fetal monitor and you will receive a Pitocin (oxytocin) injection. If the baby cannot maintain his heartbeat during a contraction, immediate delivery may be indicated (possibly by C-section).

Biophysical Profile (BPP)

A biophysical profile (BPP) is simply an ultrasound combined with a nonstress test (NST). A BPP assesses fetal heart rate, muscle tone, body and breathing movement, and the amount of amniotic fluid, which are all noted and included on your chart. The test takes about a half hour, and a score of 8 to 10 is normal. A low BPP score may indicate that the fetus is getting insufficient oxygen. If the fetal lungs are mature, immediate delivery may be recommended.

Women in high-risk pregnancies may undergo regular weekly or biweekly BPP testing in the third trimester. BPP is also a standard test for a post-term pregnancy that has gone beyond forty-two weeks. Your physician may also order a modified biophysical profile, which is a BPP that consists of the NST and an ultrasound assessment of amniotic fluid (the amniotic fluid index, or AFI) only.

Chapter 6

Woe Is Me: Those Little Aches and Pains

Have you always had visions of being a glowing, gorgeous version of yourself when you were pregnant? It's true, there is a lot that's beautiful about being pregnant—your skin looks clearer, your hair seems thicker—and who isn't awed by the amazing sight of that new life growing inside you day by day? But let's not kid ourselves here—some minor discomforts also go with the territory. Whether morning sickness stops you in your tracks from the get go, or you cruise through the first two trimesters with ease, only to be saddled with shockingly swollen ankles during phase three, you're going to have some lousy side effects to contend with. Knowing what to expect and how to combat these minor discomforts will help you to enjoy your pregnancy more and keep your life on track.

The Dreaded Monster: Morning Sickness

Beats us why anybody ever thought to call that nagging feeling of nausea—and the vomiting that sometimes accompanies it—"morning sickness," because it has no problem occurring *anytime* of the day. Every woman's experience with morning sickness is different. Some women hardly have any morning sickness at all, while others feel sick as dogs for weeks on end. (Don't worry, either way is totally normal and has no bearing on the health of your baby!) For most women, morning sickness begins in the fifth to sixth week from the first day of the last menstrual period (about the third week of pregnancy). Then it typically begins to subside around fourteen to sixteen weeks.

Like so many other things, you can blame morning sickness on—you guessed it—all those crazy hormonal changes happening in your body. In particular, the pregnancy hormone HCG (human chorionic gonadotropin) and the change in estrogen are thought to be the culprits. Take heart—although there's no way of totally getting around morning sickness if it strikes, your lifestyle can affect its severity for better or worse. Be sure to rest up, because women who don't get enough rest sometimes have a rougher time. Excess stress can exacerbate the problem, too, so stay as cool as possible.

················· **need to know** ·····················

Severe morning sickness, called hyperemesis gravidarum, can cause weight loss, dehydration, ketone production (which is toxic to a fetus), and potassium deficiency. If your morning sickness becomes severe, be sure to let your doctor know.

Testing might be done to rule out possible health conditions such as gastroenteritis, thyroid disease, cholecystitis (gall bladder), pancreatitis, hepatitis, ulcer, kidney disease, and fatty-liver disease as well as obstetric conditions such as multiple births and molar pregnancies.

Here are some other quick tips to help battle morning sickness:

- Stay away from foods with strong odors or flavors that might trigger nausea. Pregnant women sometimes develop an exaggerated sense of smell, which makes common odors unappealing.
- Keep your kitchen well ventilated during cooking and meal times.
- Let someone else do the cooking for you! (You deserve a break, after all!)
- Go easy on spicy foods.
- Before getting out of bed in the morning, eat a starchy food to help absorb and neutralize stomach acid. Carbohydrate-rich foods can help to elevate your blood-sugar levels slowly and prevent symptoms of nausea.
- Get up out of bed slowly. Standing up abruptly can make you feel dizzier and more nauseous.
- Instead of three large meals, eat five or six small meals or snacks per day every two to three hours. Usually, nausea gets worse when your stomach gets empty, so don't let yourself get too hungry—nibble on healthy snacks.
- Stay well hydrated! If it gets hard to drink beverages with meals because your stomach feels too full, do most of your drinking between meals.
- Limit fried, greasy, and other high-fat foods. Aside from being unhealthy (which should not be news to you at this point) they can be hard to digest. Stick to easy-to-digest foods like plain pasta, potatoes, rice, fruits, vegetables, lean meats, fish, poultry, and eggs.

- Eat your meals and snacks slowly.
- Before you go to bed at night, eat a light snack—peanut butter on bread and a glass of milk, yogurt, or cereal.
- Experiment with drinks that can settle a queasy stomach: lemon or ginger tea, ginger ale, lemonade, peppermint tea, or water with a slice of lemon. Some women do better with hot liquids, while others do better with cold.
- Choose foods that agree with you, and stay away from those that don't. And take heart if at first you're not able to eat the perfect balance of all those food groups you're supposed to. At least you'll be getting some food into you. Soon enough, when morning sickness passes, you can make up for lost nutrition time.
- Take advantage of the times when you do feel good, and fuel up on nutritious foods then!
- Make sure to take your iron supplements and prenatal vitamins with food, because they can sometimes intensify nausea. If your supplements are making you sick, don't stop taking them—talk to your doctor or midwife first.
- Some women say that sucking on "fireballs," those intense cinnamon jawbreakers, eases their morning sickness. Hey, it's worth a shot!

If you're having a really rough time making it through the day because of your morning sickness, speak up! Let your family know how you're feeling, and don't be shy about asking for their help and support. A little relief at home could go a long way toward helping you to rest up and destress, so you can get past your morning sickness.

Tummy Troubles—and Then Some

As if morning sickness wasn't enough . . . there are several other gastro-intestinal complaints that can leave more than just your belly grumbling during pregnancy. Once again, though, the way you eat and your lifestyle can go a long way toward relieving some of these problems.

Cranky Over Constipation

Constipation often goes with the pregnancy territory. All those hormonal changes going on help your muscles to relax. That's a good thing when it comes to accommodating your expanding uterus and making your hips and pelvis more flexible. But it's not so great when it slows the action in your intestines and the movement of food through your digestive tract. Iron in prenatal vitamins can also cause constipation. Not to mention that all the increased pressure on your intestinal tract as the baby grows can also cause hemorrhoids. Preventing constipation (as much as possible, anyway) can help you to steer clear of hemorrhoids. Hormonal changes and all that pressure from your growing baby can't be helped, but there are plenty of things you can do that will make a difference.

············ **need to know** ············

A high-fiber diet helps. (Women under fifty should shoot for twenty-five grams of fiber daily.) Eat plenty of whole-wheat breads and pastas, high-fiber breakfast cereals, bran, vegetables, fruits, and legumes.

Some foods act as natural laxatives, such as prunes, prune juice, and figs; other dried fruits might help as well. Be sure to drink plenty of fluids, though, or this could make your constipation worse. You need eight to twelve cups of fluid daily (not caffeinated drinks, which can be dehydrating). Drink mostly water, but include fruit juice and milk, too. Regular physical activity can also help to get things going where bowel function is concerned. If nothing seems to help, ask your doctor about possibly taking a fiber supplement such as bran, Metamucil, or a similar product mixed with water or juice once a day.

Laxatives are a last resort. Don't use over-the-counter laxatives or stool softeners unless you have talked to your doctor first. Some might not be safe to use during pregnancy. And avoid castor oil as a remedy because it can interfere with your body's ability to absorb some nutrients. Before turning to medications to relieve your symptoms, first make sure your diet, fluid intake, and activity level is adequate.

How Gas-tly

The same changes in a pregnant woman's body that cause constipation can also cause excess gassiness. In this case, up your fiber intake slowly and drink plenty of fluids each day. Increasing fiber too quickly, especially when you are used to a lower-fiber diet, can cause gas and other gastrointestinal problems. Some foods can exacerbate gas problems, such as broccoli, beans, cabbage, onions, cauliflower, and fried foods. Carbonated drinks also cause problems. Every woman's body is different when it comes to tolerating certain foods, so keep track of what bothers you and then cut back on those things.

Oh, the Heartburn

Heartburn has nothing to do with your heart but everything to do with your stomach and esophagus. In the beginning stages of pregnancy, hormonal changes are usually what cause heartburn. That irritated feeling and the sour taste in your mouth comes from acidic stomach juices backing up into your esophagus. As your pregnancy progresses, your growing baby puts more and more pressure on your stomach and other digestive organs, which can also cause heartburn. Although heartburn can happen any time during pregnancy, the last three months—when the baby is rapidly growing—are what really get you. Here's what you can do to help relieve heartburn:

- Eat small, frequent meals throughout the day, every hour or two if possible. (You already know this routine, thanks to morning sickness.)
- Steer clear of caffeine, chocolate, highly seasoned foods, high-fat foods, citrus fruits or juices, tomato-based products, and carbonated beverages— these offenders are known to cause heartburn.
- Keep a food diary to track foods that might be triggering your heartburn.
- Eat slowly and in a relaxed atmosphere.
- Do not lie down right after a meal; stay seated upright for an hour or two after eating. Even better, take a walk after you eat to help get your gastric juices flowing in the right direction.

- Avoid large meals before bedtime.
- Drink fluids between meals instead of with meals.
- Sleep with your head elevated to help prevent acid backup.
- Wear comfortable, loose-fitting clothing.
- Talk to your doctor about which antacids are safe to use before taking any over-the-counter medications.

Why Won't My Head Stop Pounding?

Headaches—especially tension headaches—can be common in pregnancy, particularly during the first trimester. If headaches have plagued you in the past, they might get worse during pregnancy. Though experts aren't sure why this is true, those crazy hormone levels coupled with changes in your blood circulation could be to blame. Other culprits can include quitting your caffeine habit too abruptly, lack of sleep, fatigue, allergies, eyestrain, stress, depression, hunger, or dehydration.

> **pregnancy treat**
>
> The good news is, for most women, headaches during pregnancy will probably lessen—and maybe even disappear—by the second trimester.

That's when the sudden rise in hormones stabilizes, and your body gets used to its altered chemistry. Though most headaches during pregnancy are harmless, some can indicate a more serious problem. In the second or third trimester, a headache can be the sign of preeclampsia, a serious pregnancy-induced condition that includes high blood pressure, protein in the urine, and other indicators. Your healthcare provider will monitor you very closely for this condition, but let her know if you're having serious headaches.

················· **need to know** ·······················

Treating headaches with medicine can be tricky during pregnancy. Most commonly used headache medications, such as aspirin and ibuprofen, aren't recommended for use during pregnancy.

Acetaminophen, or Tylenol, is safe to take but only as directed. Instead of medication, try other remedies first, such as a warm or cold compress applied to the forehead or back of the neck.

Headache Relief

Pinpointing the trigger of your headache can help you to relieve it. If you are in a hot, stuffy room, get some fresh air. And it's not hard to figure out if your screaming kids are making your head pound, you should probably drop them off with a relative or friend so you can get a break. Since low blood sugar can trigger headaches, keep your stomach full. Eat small meals every few hours so you don't get too hungry. Steer clear of too much sugar, which can cause blood sugar to rapidly spike and crash. If possible, take daily naps to keep fatigue at bay. Regular sleep patterns can help to reduce headaches.

Regular exercise can also help decrease the stress that sometimes causes tension headaches. Relaxation techniques incorporated into your daily routine, such as meditation and yoga, can also be helpful in reducing stress and headaches. Talk to a professional who can show you which yoga poses and other relaxation techniques are safe and helpful during pregnancy.

···················· **pregnancy treat** ····················

Pampering yourself with a warm shower or bath can go a long way toward alleviating the headache battle. Even better, if you have the time and money, get a professional to give you a massage and work out all those knots!

Managing Migraines

Migraines are fairly common in women of childbearing age. About two-thirds of women who get them before becoming pregnant notice improvement after the first trimester. This is especially true if their migraines were normally caused by hormonal changes during their menstrual cycle. Unfortunately, though, others notice no change, and some even get more frequent and intense headaches.

Migraines are a far cry from tension headaches. A migraine is a vascular headache that happens when the blood vessels in the brain constrict and then dilate rapidly. Some people have visual disturbances before the headache occurs. The pain—usually severe throbbing—is often concentrated on one side of the head. Some people also experience nausea and vomiting as well as sensitivity to light and noise. Since not much is known about what causes migraines, the best approach is to try to avoid getting one.

If you've had migraines before, you won't be able to take the same medication now that you're pregnant. Talk to your doctor right away about what's safe to take so you know ahead of time what to do. When a migraine does hit, try to sleep it off in a quiet, dark room and apply a cold compress to your forehead or neck. A cold shower can help to constrict the dilated blood vessels. If you can't take a shower, at least splash some cool water on your face and the back of your neck.

Certain foods can trigger migraines. Top offenders include foods with MSG, red wine, cured meats, chocolate, aged cheese, and preserved meats such as hot dogs or bologna. As with other headaches, low blood sugar can also trigger migraines, so keep your stomach full and your blood sugar level up. And, as mentioned earlier for headaches in general, stay active, get plenty of rest, stick to regular sleep patterns, and incorporate some stress-relieving techniques into your daily routine.

What's Going on with My Mouth?

You might freak out the first time you finish brushing your teeth, rinse out your mouth, and see blood in the sink. Don't worry too much—because of the hormonal changes that affect the blood supply to the mouth and gums, pregnancy can be demanding on your teeth, making you more susceptible to mouth and gum discomfort as well as minor bleeding. Gingivitis is especially common during the second to eighth months of pregnancy and can cause red, puffy, or tender gums that tend to bleed when you brush your teeth.

Don't Neglect Your Teeth

You might not be thinking a lot about your teeth right now, but it's important to see your dentist early in your pregnancy and keep up with checkups. Brush your teeth and tongue at least twice per day, and floss regularly. Chew sugarless gum after meals if you are not able to brush. Make sure you are taking your prenatal vitamins and calcium supplements as directed, to help strengthen your teeth and keep your mouth healthy. If you have any mouth or gum problems that are really bothersome, see your dentist so they don't interfere with eating a healthy diet.

> ### ⋯⋯⋯ need to know ⋯⋯⋯
>
> Flouride is important as baby's teeth develop. There is no need to take a supplement as long as you drink or cook with fluoridated tap water. (Bottled water usually doesn't contain fluoride.)

Also, although fluoride is not widely found in food, you can get it from tea, especially if brewed with fluoridated water, fish with edible bones, kale, spinach, apples, and nonfat milk.

The Pain That Wakes You Up
in the Middle of the Night

No, we don't mean *that* pain. At least not yet, anyway. We're talking about those pesky muscle cramps—especially leg cramps—that can plague a pregnant woman mercilessly. They usually surface in the second and third trimester of pregnancy, and they can occur at any time of day, although they get you mostly at night.

The truth is, no one really knows exactly why women get leg cramps during pregnancy. It probably has something to do with fatigue in muscles from carrying around all that extra weight. Some believe inactivity or lack of fluids is to blame. Others zero in on excess phosphorus and too little calcium, potassium, and/or magnesium in the blood. Although there's no concrete evidence that supplementing with these minerals decreases leg cramps during pregnancy, some doctors might prescribe them anyway. Your best strategy is to make sure you're getting plenty of these nutrients by eating a healthy, well-balanced diet. Don't take any additional supplements unless you've talked with your doctor. But enough about what *might* cause these nasty cramps. What you really need to know is how to steer clear of them and alleviate them when they strike. Here goes:

- Avoid standing or sitting in the same position for long periods of time. That includes sitting with your legs crossed, which can decrease blood circulation in your legs.

- Stretch your calf muscles periodically during the day and especially before going to bed at night and when waking up in the morning.
- Take a walk or do some other physical activity every day (with your doctor's permission) to help blood flow in your legs and extremities.
- Stay well hydrated—eight to twelve glasses of water daily is a must.
- Get plenty of calcium in your diet through food and prescribed supplements. Aim for three servings of dairy foods per day.
- If you get a cramp, massage the troubled area or apply a hot water bottle or heating pad to your leg. Straighten your leg and flex your ankle and toes slowly up toward your nose. If the cramp hits while you're in bed, try to stand up on it as soon as you can, because stretching the muscles this way often helps.

Just don't go overboard with calcium. Too much calcium and phosphorus might decrease the absorption of magnesium, which could also be needed to prevent muscle cramps. Too much calcium over an extended period of time can also inhibit absorption of iron and zinc as well as cause other problems.

Desperate for Sleep

Sometimes, pregnant women just can't win. You might be exhausted during the day, only to find yourself fighting sleeplessness at night. Endless trips to the bathroom because you need to pee all the time, symptoms of morning sickness, excitement, anxiety, and worrying about becoming a new mother are all normal things that can disrupt your typical sleep patterns during pregnancy. Add increased physical discomfort during the third trimester, courtesy of your now enormous abdomen, heartburn, backaches, and leg cramps, and restful sleep might seem like a fleeting memory.

If insomnia is getting to you, it might help to take afternoon naps—but not so many that it actually makes for more problems when it comes time to sleep at night. Drinking warm milk before bedtime always does the trick, and a warm bath before you sack out can help, too. Find ways to relax yourself to sleep, such as yoga, meditation, guided imagery, or reading before bedtime. Make sure your bedroom is at a comfortable temperature and it's dark and quiet. Exercise during the day can also help to settle you down for sleep. And don't take sleeping pills or other herbal remedies without talking to your doctor first.

Above all, don't get all worked up about not being able to get to sleep. That will only exacerbate the problem!

woe is me: those little aches and pains

Chapter 7

Health Beat

$\mathcal{N}$ow that you are pregnant, you want to make sure that everything you put in your mouth is safe for you and your baby. There are many different products that fall into this group, including everything from food additives to medications. Also, there are special conditions that you may be at risk to develop now that you are pregnant.

Something Fishy

Fish and seafood can be a valuable source of nutrition. Fish contains protein, omega-3 fatty acids, vitamin D, and other essential nutrients that make it an exceptionally healthy food for pregnant mothers and developing babies. However, some fish can contain harmful levels of methylmercury, a toxic mercury compound.

Harmful Effects

If consumed regularly by women who can become pregnant, women who are pregnant or nursing, or by a young child, methylmercury can harm a developing brain and nervous system. Just about all types of fish contain trace amounts of methylmercury, which is not harmful to most humans. However, larger fish that feed on other fish accumulate the highest levels of methylmercury. These types of fish pose the greatest risks to people that consume them on a regular basis.

.... **need to know** ....

Pregnant women as well as women who are trying to conceive, nursing mothers, and young children are advised to also avoid these types of fish in large amounts. Check with your physician about specific fish you should avoid eating.

Drugs to Take and to Avoid

Some pills you pop, whether prescription or over-the-counter, may have dire consequences for your developing baby. Never assume anything is safe to take unless you speak to your doctor first.

Prescription Medications

There is much controversy and plenty of gray area when it comes to the safety of prescription medications and pregnancy. There is no definitive answer on whether many medications are safe to use during pregnancy or not. Many do not have extensive, long-term studies that can give us clear-cut answers. The reality is that women can get sick during pregnancy, and many enter pregnancy with chronic conditions that require treatment with prescription medications.

Many medications cannot be stopped abruptly without adverse effects and must be discontinued gradually. It is absolutely vital that you speak with your doctor about all prescription medications you may be taking before you begin trying to conceive. Some medications that your doctor prescribed before you became pregnant may not be safe once you become pregnant. The bottom line is that all decisions regarding drug treatment during pregnancy should be made and monitored by your doctor.

Over-the-Counter Medications

Many over-the-counter products can be used safely during pregnancy under your doctor's supervision, but many can also be unsafe. Extensive testing is required for any drug before it can be labeled safe for use during pregnancy. The FDA ranking system categorizes all drugs.

Comprehensive, evidence-based guidelines for determining the safety of over-the-counter medications during pregnancy are not yet available.

Ideally, any woman taking medication during pregnancy would be under the supervision of her doctor. Over-the-counter medications should not be used unless the benefits clearly outweigh the risks.

Seek alternative methods of relieving headaches, pains, and other problems before taking an over-the-counter medication. And, as always, consult your doctor before using any over-the-counter medication regardless of what you are taking them for.

.... **need to know** ....

Take the best care of yourself by seeking prenatal care, eating a healthy diet, and being physically active to decrease your chances of becoming ill or developing such problems as constipation.

Herbal and All-Natural Supplements

There are hundreds of herbal and botanical supplements on the market today. Many pregnant women who wouldn't consider taking over-the-counter medications feel that herbal and botanical products are "natural" or "organic" and therefore safe. Never assume that just because a supplement is labeled "natural" or "organic" and is sold over the counter that it is safe to take during pregnancy. Little is known about the effects of herbal, botanical, and dietary supplements on a growing fetus and whether they are safe to use during pregnancy.

health beat

The herbs that are most indicative of possibly causing harm during pregnancy include aloe, chamomile, black cohosh, blue cohosh, devil's claw root, dong quai, ephedra, eucalyptus, fenugreek, feverfew, ginseng, guarana, hawthorne, juniper, licorice, St. John's Wort, and willow. Again, this is only a sampling of some herbal supplements that may not be safe; there are hundreds more on the market. You should check out each one, and speak to your doctor before taking any.

> ### need to know
>
> Although you should question all herbal and botanical supplements, a few popular herbs are suspected in particular of being harmful during pregnancy.

Health Concerns During Pregnancy

Though pregnancy is a happy and exciting time, health concerns can surface. It is important to understand what health problems can develop and to know the signs and symptoms to look for. You should always contact your doctor if you have signs and/or symptoms that seem abnormal to you or if you just are not feeling right. Listen to your body, and be aware of potential problems.

Hyperemesis Gravidarum

The majority of pregnant women experience some form of mild nausea and/or vomiting early in pregnancy. In fact, almost 50 percent of women experience some form of morning sickness. However, a very small percentage of women experience extremely severe and persistent nausea and/or vomiting. This is a condition known as hyperemesis gravidarum (HG). This condition can make it difficult for a mother to consume the number of calories she needs, get enough fluids, and simply perform daily activities. If this condition is left untreated, it can lead to malnutrition, vitamin and mineral deficiencies, electrolyte imbalances, weight loss, dehydration, and even possible liver or kidney damage. These symptoms can all be damaging to the development of the fetus as well as to the health of the mother. When HG is treated properly, any adverse outcome to the baby—such as low birth weight, developmental problems, or prematurity—can be avoided.

Diagnosing

Hyperemesis gravidarum is typically diagnosed through a thorough health exam, blood test, urine test, detailed health history, and the identification of symptoms characteristic to the condition including severe and persistent nausea and vomiting as well as dehydration and weight loss. HG is only considered as the final diagnosis when all other possible causes of severe and persistent nausea and vomiting have been ruled out. The condition typically begins in the period from weeks four to six and peaks between weeks nine and thirteen. Some women see significant improvements between weeks fourteen and twenty, while others may need significant care throughout the pregnancy.

Treatment

If you are diagnosed with hyperemesis gravidarum, you may need hospitalization to restore fluids, replace electrolytes, and to administer medications if needed. Some treatment plans may also include vitamin and mineral supplementation. Depending on the doctor, you may not be given food by mouth until the vomiting stops and dehydration has been rectified. Instead, your food will be supplied through a feeding tube, and you will begin on food slowly. Proper nutritional intake is one of the biggest challenges and most important issues for women who suffer from HG.

····················· **need to know** ·····················

If you are not getting sufficient nutrients to meet your baby's requirements, your baby will take it from your stores.

This can deplete your nutritional reserves very quickly, and it might take months or even years for you to correct these deficiencies. Vitamins, especially the B vitamins, can be depleted very quickly, and if they are not replaced can worsen the symptoms. With hospitalization, you can get the proper care that is needed.

Iron Deficiency Anemia

Anemia is defined as a deficiency of red blood cells or red blood cells having a decreased ability to carry oxygen or iron. There are different forms of anemia, such as iron, B12, and folate deficiency. During pregnancy, the most common is iron deficiency anemia.

It is important to be tested for anemia during your first prenatal visit so that measures can be taken for treatment if you are found to be anemic. Even if you test negative for anemia at your first visit, the condition can develop as you progress through your pregnancy.

Diagnosing

A diagnostic blood test that indicates hemoglobin and hematocrit levels can help to diagnose anemia. If these levels indicate a problem, additional blood tests and other evaluation measures may be used to properly diagnose you. Possible complications that can occur if anemia is not treated include premature labor, slowing of fetal growth, complications of dangerous anemia from normal blood loss during delivery, and an increased susceptibility of infection to the mother after delivery.

Most women are provided with iron through prenatal supplements before and during pregnancy to help prevent iron deficiency. Eating iron-rich foods such as lean meats, fortified breakfast cereals, spinach, pumpkin seeds, beans, and dried fruits can also be very helpful.

Women at higher risk of anemia are those who are unable to eat a balanced diet due to morning sickness or hyperemesis gravidarum, who are pregnant with multiple babies, and who have overall poor eating habits, including inadequate iron intake. Your iron needs increase by 50 percent in pregnancy due to an increase in blood volume. Especially if your iron stores were not optimal before becoming pregnant, your iron can easily get used up to meet the demands of pregnancy, and that can lead to the risk of anemia. Good nutrition and proper supplementation before becoming pregnant and during pregnancy is vital to help build up your stores of iron and prevent the risk of iron deficiency anemia.

Signs and Symptoms

Unless blood cell counts are very low, the signs and symptoms of anemia can be very subtle. Symptoms vary from person to person and depend on the severity of the condition. Some symptoms include fatigue and weakness, headache, dizziness, rapid heartbeat, pale skin, and labored breathing or breathlessness.

Symptoms of anemia can closely resemble those of other health conditions and/or medical problems. Never diagnose or treat yourself. Always consult your doctor for a proper diagnosis.

Gestational Diabetes

Gestational diabetes mellitus (GDM) is a type of diabetes, or insulin resistance, that develops around the middle of pregnancy and ends after delivery. Women who are pregnant, have high blood sugar (glucose) levels, and have never had diabetes before are said to have GDM. Gestational diabetes occurs when the body isn't able to properly use insulin or to make enough insulin to keep blood sugar levels in normal ranges, causing higher-than-normal levels. Without enough insulin, or with the body not using it properly, glucose cannot leave the blood and be used for energy. GDM usually develops around the sixth month of pregnancy, or between the twenty-fourth and twenty-eighth weeks.

It can be unhealthy for both mother and baby if blood sugar levels are too high. Because GDM does not appear until later in the pregnancy when the baby has been formed, it does not cause birth defects seen in some babies whose mothers had diabetes before pregnancy.

························· **need to know** ·······················

If GDM is not treated properly or controlled, it can cause problems for the baby that include low blood sugar levels, jaundice, breathing problems, and high insulin levels.

In addition, it can cause a baby to weigh more than normal at birth, which can make delivery more difficult and possibly necessitate a cesarean section. Babies born with excess insulin run a higher risk of obesity in childhood and adulthood, thereby putting them at higher risk for Type 2 diabetes later in life. GDM is different from other forms of diabetes in that it only occurs during pregnancy and goes away after delivery. Women who have diabetes before becoming pregnant are not classified as having gestational diabetes.

Some women do not experience any symptoms with gestational diabetes. Therefore, it is standard practice to screen most pregnant women at the

health beat

twenty-eighth week of pregnancy. Women who are high risk for GDM are screened at their first doctor's visit as well as at twenty-eight weeks.

Causes

Gestational diabetes seems to stem from the placenta and its production of several hormones that help the baby develop during pregnancy. During the second and third trimesters, these "insulin-antagonist" hormone levels increase and can cause insulin resistance. Insulin resistance makes it difficult for the mother's body to properly utilize insulin, the hormone that manages glucose or blood sugar levels. This causes a higher-than-normal blood sugar level, or hyperglycemia. After delivery, these hormone levels, as well as glucose levels, return to normal.

Some women are at higher risk than others for developing gestational diabetes. Among this group are women with a strong family history of diabetes or a first-degree relative with diabetes, women who are obese, women who have had problem pregnancies in the past, women with a history of having babies more than nine pounds at birth, women who have had gestational diabetes in past pregnancies, and women over the age of twenty-five. Also counted as high risk are women of certain ethnicities, including African-Americans, Latinos, Asian-Americans, Native Americans, and Pacific Islanders.

Treatment

If you are diagnosed with gestational diabetes, treatment needs to begin immediately. The goal of treatment is to help keep blood sugar levels within a safe range to help reduce the risk of complications to you and your baby during pregnancy and after delivery. Most women are able to keep their blood sugar levels within a safe range by eating a well-balanced diet that balances carbohydrates (55 to 60 percent of calories), protein, and fat. Regular exercise can also help to keep blood sugar levels in balance. Treatment should also include daily blood glucose testing. If a balanced diet and regular exercise are not enough to help control blood sugar levels, insulin injections may be needed. Oral glucose medications are not recommended during pregnancy.

Hypertension and Preeclampsia

High blood pressure, or hypertension, occurs when there is a consistently higher-than-normal pressure or force of blood against the walls of your arteries. It is normal for a pregnant woman's blood pressure to drop during her first and second trimesters. By the third trimester, however, blood pressure usually returns to normal levels. However, in about 8 to 10 percent of pregnant women, instead of returning to normal, blood pressure begins to increase to abnormally high levels in the second or third trimester. This condition is known as pregnancy-induced hypertension. Women who enter pregnancy with high blood pressure are said to have chronic high blood pressure.

Preeclampsia, which is also sometimes called toxemia, is a disorder that only occurs during pregnancy and can also occur during the period right after delivery. It can greatly affect both the mother and unborn baby.

health beat

Preeclampsia occurs in about 5 to 8 percent of all pregnancies, and very severe cases of preeclampsia can be life threatening. Typically, this condition develops after the twentieth week of pregnancy, in the late second trimester and into the third trimester, although for some it can develop earlier. High blood pressure that develops before the twentieth week is usually a sign of chronic high blood pressure or pregnancy-induced hypertension, but it can also be an early sign of preeclampsia.

··········· **need to know** ···········

Mild hypertension during pregnancy is not necessarily dangerous by itself, but it can be a sign of a more serious condition called preeclampsia. High blood pressure puts a woman at higher risk for preeclampsia.

Untreated, preeclampsia can cause high blood pressure, problems with blood supply to the placenta and fetus, problems to the liver, kidney, and brain function of the mother as well as the risk of stroke, seizures, and fluid on the lungs. Because the condition affects the blood flow to the placenta and fetus, the baby has a harder time getting the oxygen and nourishment it needs. These babies are often smaller in size and tend to be born prematurely. Women who develop severe preeclampsia can develop life-threatening seizures called eclampsia.

There is no single test that can diagnose preeclampsia. Your blood pressure is checked at each and every doctor's visit, which makes regular prenatal care even more essential for all pregnant women. A sudden rise in your blood pressure can be an early sign of preeclampsia. A urine test is also used to check for protein in the urine, which can be another warning sign.

High blood pressure does not necessarily mean you have preeclampsia. In addition to high blood pressure, women with preeclampsia tend to have excessive swelling or edema in the hands and face as well as protein in the urine. Many women who experience high blood pressure during pregnancy without these other symptoms don't have preeclampsia.

Causes

The causes of high blood pressure and/or preeclampsia are not actually known. Preeclampsia seems to have a possible genetic link because women with a family history of the condition have a higher risk than those who do not. Preeclampsia is more common in first pregnancies as well. Other factors that put women at a higher risk include high blood pressure, diabetes, an autoimmune disease such as lupus, or a kidney disorder before pregnancy.

Signs and Symptoms

The signs and symptoms of pregnancy-induced hypertension and preeclampsia can be classified into three categories: mild, moderate, and severe. The signs and symptoms of high blood pressure and preeclampsia are often silent if the condition is mild. Suspicions usually surface unexpectedly during routine blood pressure checks and urine tests. Moderate preeclampsia can bring with it signs of high blood pressure, protein in the urine, rapid weight gain (more than one pound a day), problems with blood clotting, and excessive swelling of the hands and face.

> ················· **need to know** ·······················
>
> Severe preeclampsia can show signs of brain or certain body organ trouble, such as severe headaches, dizziness, vision problems, breathing problems, abdominal pain, and decreased urination.

Very rarely, preeclampsia can progress to a condition called eclampsia that can be life threatening, especially if the preeclampsia is not treated properly and early enough.

Treatment

If you are diagnosed with preeclampsia, treatment depends on the severity of your condition, the health of your baby, and the stage of your pregnancy. It is recommended that you lie on your left side as much as possible to help take unnecessary pressure off the blood vessels. This allows for greater blood flow.

If you develop mild preeclampsia close to your due date, and your cervix is showing signs of thinning and dilation, your doctor may want to induce labor. This will help prevent any complications that could develop if the preeclampsia were to worsen before your delivery.

If your cervix is not showing signs that it is ready for induction, your doctor will probably monitor you and your baby very closely until the time is right to induce or until labor begins on its own. If you develop preeclampsia before the thirty-seventh week of pregnancy, your doctor will most likely recommend bed rest, either at home or in the hospital, depending on your situation. For some, depending on the severity of the blood pressure, blood pressure medication will be prescribed until the pressure stabilizes or until delivery. With severe preeclampsia, a medication to prevent eclampsia (a very serious condition involving seizures) may also be prescribed.

Even though cutting salt from your diet is usually a good way to help control high blood pressure, it is not a good idea to cut the salt in your diet if you have high blood pressure during pregnancy. It is essential that your body gets a normal intake of salt during pregnancy. Ask your doctor and a registered dietitian for advice and information.

In general, if you develop preeclampsia, delivery of your baby is the best way to protect you both from complications. If this isn't possible because it is too early in the pregnancy, steps will be taken to manage the preeclampsia until your baby can be safely delivered and survive outside of the womb.

At this point, early diagnosis through simple blood pressure checks and other routine tests at regular prenatal visits is the best way to detect pregnancy-induced hypertension or preeclampsia. The earlier the condition is detected, the earlier treatment and monitoring can begin and the better chance you and your baby have for a healthy pregnancy and healthy delivery.

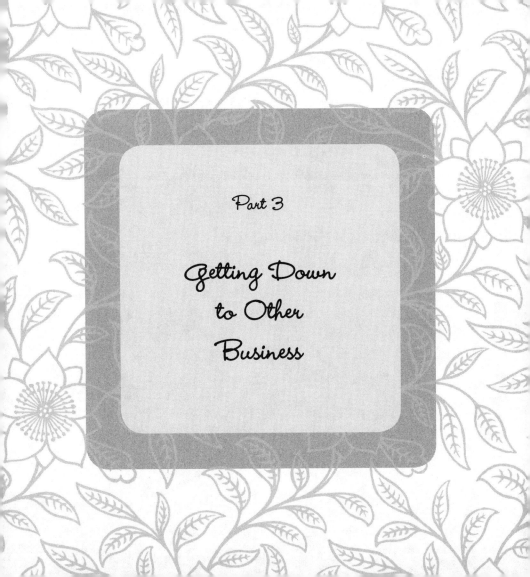

Part 3

Getting Down
to Other
Business

Chapter 8

You Are What You Eat

There is much to learn about how to properly nourish yourself and your growing baby. This chapter will help you eat your way through a healthy pregnancy. Please note that the intake requirements and recommended daily allowances described in this chapter are for women aged nineteen to fifty. Women outside this range may have slightly different requirements.

Focus on Folic Acid

Folate, found naturally in foods, is one of the B vitamins; it is also known as folic acid, which is the name for the form found in supplements and fortified foods. Folic acid merits special consideration. During pregnancy, this vitamin helps to properly develop the neural tube, which becomes the baby's spine. When taken in daily optimal amounts at least one month before becoming pregnant and during the first trimester, folic acid can help prevent birth defects of the brain and spinal cord, called neural tube defects (NTDs).

Though the Institute of Medicine of the National Academies still states that the recommended intake is 400 mcg for women of childbearing age, recent studies show that to decrease the risk of birth defects, folic acid should be increased to 800 to 1000 mcg daily (the amount in most prenatal vitamins) in those attempting pregnancy. So your doctor will likely prescribe a prenatal vitamin with this higher amount.

Spina bifida, sometimes called "open spine," affects the backbone and sometimes the spinal cord. Spina bifida is the most common severe birth defect in the United States, affecting 1,500 to 2,000 babies (1 in every 2,000 live births) each year. Anencephaly is a fatal condition in which the baby is born with a severely underdeveloped brain and skull.

Because most women do not know that they are pregnant right away and because the neural tube and the brain begin to form so quickly after conception, taking optimal amounts of folic acid on a daily basis is important for all women in their childbearing years.

Intake Requirements

Even though a woman follows a healthy, well-balanced diet, she may still not be consuming the recommended amount of folic acid each day. For this reason, in 1998 the Institute of Medicine recommended "that to reduce their risk for an NTD-affected pregnancy, women capable of becoming pregnant should take at least 400 mcg of synthetic folic acid daily, from fortified foods or supplements or a combination of the two, in addition to consuming food folate from a varied diet." You can use an over-the-counter multivitamin/mineral supplement or prenatal supplement to make sure you get your folic acid. Check the label on over-the-counter supplements because not all contain folic acid in the recommended amounts. The intake for folate increases with pregnancy and breastfeeding. Women who have previously had a baby with an NTD may have higher folate requirements and should speak with their doctors.

Until more information becomes available, both pregnant and nonpregnant women ages nineteen years and older should not exceed the tolerable upper limit of 1,000 mcg of folate per day from foods, fortified foods, and supplements unless otherwise prescribed by their doctor.

·················· **pregnancy treat** ··················

To help women consume more folate, in 1998 the U.S. Food and Drug Administration (FDA) required that all grain products such as breads, flour, crackers, and rice be fortified with folic acid.

Other very good sources of folate include orange juice, fortified breakfast cereals, lentils, dried beans, dark-green leafy vegetables, spinach, broccoli, peanuts, wheat germ, and avocados. Folate can be destroyed during cooking, so eat fruits and vegetables raw or cook them for as short a time as possible by steaming, microwaving, or stir-frying.

According to the U.S. Center for Disease Control (CDC), when taken one month before conception and throughout the first trimester, folic acid supplements have been proven to reduce the risk for an NTD-affected pregnancy by 50 to 70 percent.

Charge Up the Calcium

Calcium is a mineral that deserves special attention throughout a woman's life, especially when it comes to pregnancy. Calcium is important to strong bones and teeth, a healthy heart, nerves, and muscles, and the development of normal heart rhythm and blood-clotting abilities. Not consuming enough calcium and/or not having good calcium stores will force the baby to use calcium from your own bones. Consuming plenty of calcium before, during, and after pregnancy can also help to reduce your risk for osteoporosis later in life.

Intake Requirements

Whether pregnant or not, calcium needs for teens (age fourteen to eighteen) is 1,300 milligrams (mg) and 1,000 mg for woman nineteen to fifty. Women older than fifty need 1,200 mg of calcium daily. The tolerable upper intake level for calcium is 2,500 mg daily.

The easiest way to get all the calcium you need is to eat at least two to three servings of low-fat or fat-free dairy foods each day. Other sources include green leafy vegetables, calcium-fortified orange juice, calcium-fortified soy milk, fish with edible bones, and tofu made with calcium sulfate. Reading the nutrition facts panel is a great way to spot calcium-rich foods. The amount on the panel is presented in terms of "% Daily Value," which is an approximation of the percentage of your day's calcium need supplied by one serving of that food.

There are all types of calcium supplements on the market today. Ideally, a calcium supplement should also contain vitamin D for maximum absorption to occur.

Elemental Calcium

In a discussion of the amount of calcium in supplements, it is important to understand the concept of elemental calcium. Calcium occurs in combination with other substances, forming compounds such as calcium carbonate, calcium phosphate, or calcium citrate. What is really important is the "elemental" calcium, or the actual amount of calcium in the compound. Some compounds contain more elemental calcium than others. For instance, a calcium supplement made from calcium carbonate might have 625 mg in each tablet, but the amount of elemental calcium in each tablet is about 250 mg. When looking for a calcium supplement, be sure to read the label carefully. Ideally, the label will list how much elemental

you are what you eat

calcium is in each tablet. If the label does not state elemental calcium, you can figure it out with the following chart. Elemental calcium accounts for these percentages of the following compounds:

- 40 percent of calcium carbonate
- 21 percent of calcium citrate
- 13 percent of calcium lactate
- 9 percent of calcium gluconate

How to Take Calcium Supplements

Supplements that contain calcium citrate can be taken with or without food, whereas calcium carbonate should be taken with food for optimal absorption. Many antacids, such as Tums, contain calcium carbonate, which may be a more convenient and less expensive way to take your calcium. If you prefer a chewable pill, products such as Viactiv can be a good choice. Avoid the natural-source calcium pills, such as those produced from oyster shell, dolomite, or bone meal. These supplements may contain lead or other toxic metals.

············· **need to know** ·························

When taking calcium supplements, it is best to take smaller amounts several times a day for the best absorption.

If you are taking a calcium supplement and an iron supplement or a supplement with iron in it, take them at different times of the day. They will each be better absorbed alone.

Pump Up the Iron

Iron is another essential mineral that merits special attention as part of your diet before and during pregnancy. Iron is essential to the formation of healthy red blood cells, which are responsible for carrying oxygen through your blood to the cells of your body. Almost two-thirds of the iron in your body is found in hemoglobin, the protein in red blood cells that carries oxygen to your body's tissues. The increase in blood volume that takes place during pregnancy greatly increases a woman's need for iron. If you do not get enough iron and/or do not have adequate iron stores, the growing baby will take it at your expense. Iron deficiency during pregnancy can cause anemia, extreme fatigue, a low birth-weight baby, and other potential problems. The greater your iron stores before you become pregnant, the better iron will be absorbed during pregnancy.

Intake Requirements

It is very difficult to get enough iron from foods alone. Most multivitamin/mineral supplements and/or prenatal vitamin supplements will provide you with your prepregnancy needs of 18 mg per day. If you have anemia before becoming pregnant, your doctor may prescribe a much larger dose. During pregnancy, your iron requirement climbs to 27 mg per day.

Again, as with many other vitamin and minerals, too much iron is not always best. Iron has a tolerable upper intake level of 45 mg. Foods that supply iron include meat, poultry, fish, legumes, and whole-grain and enriched grain products. Iron from plant sources (or "nonheme iron") is not as easily absorbed as that from animal sources (or "heme iron"). Supplementing your meals with a food or beverage rich in vitamin C, such as citrus fruits or juices, broccoli, tomatoes, or kiwi, will help your body better absorb the iron in the foods you consume. The absorption of iron from supplements is best absorbed on an empty stomach or when swallowed with juice containing vitamin C.

The Scoop on Prenatal Vitamins

Prenatal supplements (PNVs) are specialized vitamin and mineral supplements that women can take even before pregnancy to get all of the essential nutrients they need during pregnancy. Studies have shown that the use of prenatal supplements before and throughout pregnancy can benefit a healthy baby.

Foods contain hundreds of vitamins, minerals, and phytonutrients. Only food supplies the ideal mixture of these substances that are essential for optimal health. Supplements can provide you with insurance that you will receive everything you need, but they cannot do the entire job.

Prenatal vitamins come in many formulations. Most PNV are distributed as samples to physician's offices, and it is a good idea to try multiple samples because some have stool softeners and other binders, which you may or may not tolerate. Finding one that you can tolerate will make it easier to take and therefore easier to remember to take it daily.

> ·················· **need to know** ··················
>
> Vitamins and minerals should never replace a healthy diet. They are only meant to supplement a healthy diet, not take the place of any one food or any food group.

The Ideal Prenatal Vitamin

The components all PNV supplements should have in common are folic acid, iron, and calcium. Most PNVs have only 100 to 250 mg of calcium—women need 1,000 to 1,200 mg daily, so you should also take a separate calcium supplement. Except for calcium, you should never take any additional supplements with your prenatal supplement unless they are prescribed by your doctor. Since some over-the-counter supplements contain too-high levels of vitamins and minerals, it may be smarter to use a supplement such as a PNV that has been specifically formulated for pregnant women and/or women trying to conceive.

PNVs are not recommended postpartum unless the mother is considered to be at "nutritional risk." Some women can benefit from taking prenatal vitamins postpartum if they plan to become pregnant in less than one year, but most experts recommend spacing pregnancy by at least one year.

Who Should Take Supplements?

If you are a healthy woman who eats a well-balanced diet and has no risk factors, your doctor may not feel that you need to take a prenatal supplement. This is something that you need to discuss with your doctor so together you can determine what is right for you. No matter how healthily you eat, it is generally difficult to get what you need each and every day, especially while pregnant or trying to conceive, so a prenatal supplement can act as insurance. All doctors do agree that a folic acid supplement is necessary.

Women who have a history of poor eating habits, who are on a restricted diet such as a vegan diet, or who require a specific nutrient due to an existing medical condition will definitely need to take some type of supplement.

Women who are expecting more than one baby or have closely spaced pregnancies will need extra iron and may require additional vitamin and mineral supplementation. Nourishing two babies demands more from your body and therefore requires more nutrients. After pregnancy, your body may be depleted of some nutrients. If you are planning to become pregnant again soon, you may need special supplements to restore those nutrients. Speak to your doctor before starting any supplement program.

Determining Your Caloric Needs

There are many different methods for estimating caloric needs. It is important to remember that these methods result only in estimates; still, you can get a general idea of the number of calories your body needs. Everyone's caloric needs differ, depending on factors such as age, gender, size, body composition, basal metabolic rate, and physical activity.

On average, a moderately active woman needs between 1,800 and 2,200 calories per day. A pregnant woman needs about 2,500 calories after the first trimester. However, because you don't spend every day lying in bed, you have additional calorie needs on top of your basal rate. The next section describes how to determine the number of calories you should ingest every day.

You Do the Math

Use this simple equation to figure your basic calorie needs:

1. **First, figure your basal metabolic rate to get the minimum number of calories your body needs to maintain a healthy weight.** To do this, multiply your healthy weight (in pounds) by ten. For instance, a woman whose healthy weight is 165 pounds would have a basal metabolic rate of 1,650—in other words, this

woman needs to take in a minimum of 1,650 calories to maintain her body weight.

2. **Figure how many additional calories you need to sustain your level of physical activity.** To do this, choose the activity level from the following list that best describes you and take the appropriate percentage of your basal metabolic rate.

Sedentary—You mainly engage in low-intensity activities throughout your day, such as sitting, driving a car, lying down, sleeping, standing, typing, or reading. Take 20 percent of your basal metabolic rate (multiply by 0.2).

Light activity—Your day includes light exercise, such as walking, but for no more than two hours of your day. Take 30 percent of your basal metabolic rate (multiply by 0.3).

Moderate activity—You engage in moderate exercise throughout the day, such as heavy housework, gardening, dancing, with very little sitting. Take 40 percent of your basal metabolic rate (multiply by 0.4).

High activity—You engage in active physical sports or have a labor-intensive job, such as construction work, on a daily basis. Take 50 percent of your basal metabolic rate (multiply by 0.5).

3. **Figure out how many additional calories you need to sustain your body's digestion and absorption of nutrients.** To do this,

add your results from steps 1 and 2, then take 10 percent of the total (multiply by 0.1).

4. **To find your total calorie needs, add your basal metabolic rate from step 1, the calories to sustain your level of physical activity from step 2, and the number of calories needed for digestion from step 3.** Take the example of the 165-pound woman from step 1, with the basal metabolic rate of 1,650. She is moderately active, which means she needs an additional 660 calories to sustain her activity level. She needs 231 calories to fuel her body's digestion and food absorption processes $(1,650 + 660 \times 0.1 = 231)$. Adding those values gives us a total of 2,541, which is the total number of calories a moderately active 165-pound woman should ingest to maintain her weight.

5. **To account for the additional calories you need to sustain your body weight during pregnancy, add 300 to the total from step 4.** This final value represents your estimated basic calorie needs.

The Pregnancy Food Guide Pyramid

Eating a variety of foods from all of the food groups is the best way to ensure you are getting the calories and nutrients you need. The USDA's Food Guide Pyramid is a good guideline for pregnant women; it ensures you consume the following minimum number of servings in each food group (about 2,500 calories):

- **9 servings from the bread, cereal, rice, and pasta group.** Examples of a single serving from this group include a slice of whole-wheat bread, ½ cup cooked cereal, half a bagel, or ½ cup of pasta. Be sure to include whole-grain and whole-wheat starches as well as other starches higher in fiber.

- **4 servings from the vegetable group.** Examples of a single serving from this group include 1 cup of raw leafy vegetables, ½ cup of other vegetables, raw or cooked, or ¾ cup vegetable juice. Choose a variety of vegetables—the darker the color, the more nutrients a vegetable has.

- **3 servings from the fruit group.** Examples of a single serving from this group include a medium apple, a small banana, a small orange, ½ cup chopped fruit, or ¾ cup fruit juice. Choose a variety of fruits daily, as raw fruits are higher in fiber than juices.

- **3–4 servings from the milk, yogurt, and cheese group.** Examples of a single serving from this group include 1 cup of milk or yogurt, 1.5 ounces natural cheese, or 2 ounces processed cheese. Use fat-free or low-fat milk, nonfat or low-fat yogurt, and low-fat cheese.

- **6–7 ounces (2–3 servings) from the meat, poultry, fish, dry beans, eggs, and nuts group.** Examples of a single serving from this group include 3 ounces poultry, fish, or lean meat; 1 ounce meat = ½ cup cooked dried beans, a whole egg, ½ cup tofu, ½ cup nuts, or 2 tablespoons peanut butter. Choose lean meats and trim fat from meat before cooking. With poultry, remove skin. Include cooked dry beans often as the main dish in meals.

Chapter 9

Fit as a Fiddle

$\mathcal{W}$hile the word fitness may bring to mind sweating and buff bodies, this image is not appropriate for pregnancy. Fitness during the nine months of pregnancy is more about health and wellness than at nearly any other point in your life.

In fact, many women and their families do not even start on the path to fitness until they become pregnant. This major life change alters the outlook and goals you have in nearly every respect. It is a time to re-evaluate your priorities for a healthy lifestyle.

Talking to Your Practitioner about Exercise

Talking with your doctor or midwife about exercise might seem way down on your list of things to discuss in the precious few minutes you have during a regular prenatal appointment. But you can't afford not to talk about this issue. Looking at the benefits of pregnancy exercise, you now know it is important to exercise, but it is also crucial that you receive guidance from those taking care of you during your pregnancy.

Ask your practitioner his or her opinion on exercise during pregnancy. Does she seem to agree with the current guidelines for pregnancy fitness released by the American College of Obstetricians and Gynecologists (ACOG)? If she doesn't, ask if there is a specific reason you should not exercise or should not exercise to the extent that you believe you should be able to during this pregnancy.

······················· **need to know** ·······················

A copy of the newest guidelines regarding exercise during pregnancy from the American College of Obstetricians and Gynecologists (ACOG) can be obtained by writing ACOG at *resources@acog.org*.

If she doesn't seem to have an answer that is satisfactory, ask her if she is aware of the latest guidelines from ACOG. If she is not aware, offer to share your copy.

Maybe you're one of the lucky women who has a practitioner who is very up-to-date on the latest exercise guidelines and is actually encouraging you. Perhaps your provider has a belief in exercise that exceeds the ACOG guidelines. Finding a happy medium—the middle of the road that both you and your practitioner can live with—goes both ways. Talking to your doctor or midwife will help you tailor a fitness program for you and your baby that is safe and effective. This will help ensure a healthy and safe pregnancy fitness course.

Risk Factors

There are certain risk factors that predispose you to potential complications while exercising during pregnancy. These potential happenings are usually not a problem if you take the proper precautions. The key in preparing for and preventing mishaps is to look ahead, to know changes you can expect in your pregnant body.

Center of Gravity

Your center of gravity is located in the middle of your abdomen, just above your belly button or umbilicus. Usually, you will not notice any changes to this area until you are into your third or fourth month of pregnancy. Once your uterus has begun to grow out of your pelvic region, your center of gravity will shift upward.

This shift itself is not painful, nor is it cause for alarm. In fact, you will probably not even notice the changes taking place, as it is a gradual process. Your body will naturally adapt to most center of gravity changes. What you do need to watch for is the natural loss of balance that may occur that will probably continue throughout pregnancy, steadily growing as your abdomen does.

The good news is that even a serious fall is generally not harmful to your baby. He or she is tucked safely away in the amniotic sac, blissfully unaware of your most recent belly flop. A shift in the center of gravity is more likely to cause problems with your posture as well. Posture is key to feeling good and looking good during your pregnancy. While exercising, simply be aware of your abdomen and try to remain conscious of the movements you are making and how you are moving. This awareness can help with any problems you might experience.

················· **need to know** ·························

Many women report that they feel off balance as their abdomen grows. You might experience this as well. The biggest danger is that the shift makes falls more likely.

Joints and Flexibility

As with everything in pregnancy, your joints are also affected. This includes your elbows, shoulders, hips, knees, wrists, and ankles. The usual culprits, your hormones, namely relaxin, are to blame for the increased risk of injury to these areas. Joints can be injured very easily during pregnancy. Using the warmup sessions and cooldowns, you can greatly reduce the risk of harming the joints during pregnancy. These exercises also have the added benefits of working your range of motion.

Previous Exercise Status

You can't pay enough attention to previous exercise habits during pregnancy. While it's perfectly acceptable to begin a mild exercise program if you've never exercised before, the problem is more with people who are used to exercising frequently prior to pregnancy. For these people, there is often a fear of exercising to the point of a good workout. If you've been exercising before your pregnancy, you can probably do the same workouts with only a few modifications for added safety. This is something that can be decided by taking cues from your body, your baby, and your practitioner.

The Physiological Effects

There is a lot of medical literature available on exercise in general. While everyone knows that exercise is good for you, it does not mean we all participate in it. Now that it has been established that exercise is good, even for an expectant woman, we are finding that more and more women are getting out and getting fit, or staying fit during pregnancy.

The physiological benefits of exercise on pregnancy are great. Not only can exercise change the course of your pregnancy and of your labor, but it can also help you reduce stress. The benefits also go well into the postpartum period and beyond.

Body awareness is a key component to exercise in pregnancy (and pregnancy in general!).

·············· **pregnancy treat** ··············

As you begin to exercise, your body awareness increases. This attention to your body can help you become more attuned to problems before they become larger issues.

This can in turn lead to an increase in attention to proper body mechanics and body posture, both of which are key to a comfortable pregnancy.

The goals of pregnancy fitness are to maintain the strength and wellness that you currently have, while preventing physical problems from occurring. For the woman who is already very fit this might mean actually slowing down a normal workout as the pregnancy advances. Clearly, if you are just starting a fitness program, exercise will be an increase in your activity. Though an increase in activity should not be a drastic one, as pregnancy is not the time to rebuild your body, you can still safely begin a fitness program during pregnancy. As you look at the benefits of exercising while pregnant, it is very obvious what the answer should be: just do it!

The Psychological Effects

There are many emotional and mental benefits as well to gain from exercise. It has long been shown that, in general, exercising helps to lower your stress levels. This stress reduction is very important during such a tense, albeit happy, time in your life.

The sense of confidence and self-esteem that comes from exercise helps you envision your newly rounding figure with pride and pleasure. You now see the beauty and function of your new pregnant form. This is just another benefit of knowing the body you live in.

Finally, as exercise becomes a part of your way of life, it becomes a habit, a healthy habit that can be shared as a family. Exercising moms rarely just quit exercising after the birth of their babies. They begin exercising with their babies. This starts the baby on a lifelong journey to seek out fitness for him or herself, because it is what he or she has learned by Mom's great example.

The Effects on Baby

In the past, one of the main concerns about exercise during pregnancy was that it would have a negative effect on your baby. To the contrary, researchers have now found that there are many physical and psychological benefits for a baby when Mom exercises during pregnancy.

As you become more aware of your pregnant body and your baby, you focus on taking proper care of that body and baby. By watching how and what you eat, you decrease the risks of preterm labor. The decrease in pre-term birth rates alone prevents many neonatal deaths, as preterm birth is one of the leading causes of death in newborns.

Healthier Placenta

The improved blood circulation of the mother through exercise can help grow a healthier placenta, which is the baby's lifeline during pregnancy, as it uses the placenta to get nutrients and oxygen and to expel waste products. The heartier the placenta, the healthier the baby will be.

Improved Labor Tolerance

Babies of mothers who exercise also seem to tolerate labor better. These babies are used to having Mom work hard while exercising, so that when it is time for Mom to have contractions—it is just another workout for them. This tolerance level has also shown to decrease the incidence of meconium (baby's first stool) in the amniotic fluid at birth. Having too much meconium in the amniotic fluid is potentially life threatening and something you would prefer to avoid.

Leaner, Healthier Babies

If you exercise during pregnancy, your baby will tend to be of a lower birth weight. While this might seem like a negative outcome, the lower weight is not from fetal growth restriction, but rather the reduction in deposits of unnecessary fat for the baby. These leaner babies at birth are also healthier and leaner later in life. Some studies even report that babies born to mothers who exercised during pregnancy were easier to care for after birth and seemed to adjust to their environments more readily.

Perhaps these babies are reported to be easier because the rocking motions associated with maternal exercise during pregnancy offered stimulation to enhance baby's brain development. One study, "Morphometric and neurodevelopmental outcome at age five years of the offspring of women who continued to exercise regularly throughout pregnancy" (J. Pediatr. 1996 Dec.; 129[6]:856–63), shows that these babies actually had better language and intelligence scores at five years of life.

Recent studies have shown that exercise in pregnancy is a safe and effective way to maintain a healthy pregnancy. While this has not always been the thinking, we now see the benefits to maintaining the strength and flexibility of the pregnant body. You and your baby have many benefits to gain.

How to Know When to Stop

We have all heard the "no pain, no gain" mantra that is so common in health centers today. While it is true that you have to expend energy to get the benefit of exercise, pain has no place in exercise, particularly during pregnancy.

Pain

Pain is your body's way of saying something is wrong. When you are pregnant, it is even more important that you pay attention to these signals from your body. Remember, your baby is counting on you to listen.

fit as a fiddle

Sometimes pain is a signal that you have a hurt muscle or a leg cramp. While these may not have a direct negative effect on your pregnancy, they can harm your body.

This type of cramping pain may be more likely to occur during pregnancy. For example, if you have a leg cramp, it may be a sign that your electrolytes are out of balance and that you need to watch your nutritional intake more closely or stretch more often. An injured muscle could result from your body's release of the hormone relaxin, which helps to facilitate the birth but also has the effect of making injuries more likely.

·········· **need to know** ··························

Pain should be something that makes you stop exercising immediately. No matter where the location of the pain or what the feeling is like, stop doing whatever you are doing.

Falls

Due to the changes in your center of gravity and the hormones coursing through your body, falls may be more likely when pregnant. For this reason, some exercises (e.g., horseback riding) are never recommended during pregnancy.

While you may be at an increased risk for falls, learning to take certain precautions can certainly help reduce this likelihood. During your normal daily life avoid high heels, walk on pathways whenever you can, and avoid uneven surfaces or stones. Whenever you work out, remember to wear the appropriate footwear.

If you do fall, try not to panic. Check yourself out completely before standing back up. In general, your baby is well protected by the amniotic sac in your uterus. However, if you experience any abdominal pain, bleeding, contractions, or changes in the baby's movements, report this immediately to your practitioner.

Feeling Weak or Dizzy

Feeling weak or dizzy is a sign that you probably need to skip your exercise today. These feelings can be a normal part of your pregnancy, or they may indicate a problem. Sometimes you feel weak from the exhaustion of pregnancy, more typically in the first and third trimesters. Other issues for feeling weak or dizzy would be a dramatic fluctuation in your blood sugar levels.

·········· **need to know** ··········

If you begin to feel weak or lightheaded during your workout, stop immediately. Sit down or lie down. Have someone bring you water. You should not try to drive or walk.

If you actually pass out, be sure to call your doctor or midwife as soon as you awake. Call your doctor or midwife right away if the symptoms don't go away within a few minutes. Otherwise, report your symptoms to your practitioner during normal office hours. They may suggest you alter your exercise plan going forward.

Sometimes simply not feeling right is a perfect indicator to stop. It could be you're having an off day. Maybe you've not eaten recently enough or perhaps you're tired. Whatever the reason, listen to your body and stop exercising.

What Is Your Fitness Level?

Finding your fitness level is the first step in any pregnancy or prepregnancy exercise program. By using some simple questions about your fitness level, you can then decide on the appropriate place to begin for your current pregnancy. An evaluation should be done with each pregnancy, as your fitness level will change throughout your life.

One of the most important elements of the evaluation, however, will not be which category you are in, but rather your determination and dedication to the exercise program. Remember that intermittent exercise can be more harmful to your body than no exercise at all.

When you exercise irregularly, you're always in the initial phases of exercise. You never really build up to anything, as you can't get past the initial stages of the training. There are also mental reasons why irregular exercise is harmful—because it never gets "any better." You are always doing something that feels difficult to do. This can make you lack the desire to exercise and can also make you more prone to injury.

Let's look at three main fitness levels that will help you define where you fit in: sedentary, moderately active, and athletic.

Sedentary

If you are sedentary, you probably have not been participating in any type of formal exercise program. You may not exercise at all, or very little. Just because you fit into these criteria does not mean that you are necessarily overweight or unhealthy. You might simply just not be as fit as you potentially could be.

Moderately Active

Do you consider yourself moderately active? If so, you probably enjoy exercise but do not go out of your way to make it a regular part of your life. You may exercise when it is convenient or fits into your social schedule, like a walk in the neighborhood with a friend, or a random aerobics or yoga class. You are more likely to add small portions of exercise to your life, like walking short distances rather than driving or parking in the back of the parking lot. This category is more for the social exerciser.

Athletic

You would know if you were classified as an athlete, although this category is not restricted to only professional athletes. You value your exercise highly and would be very lost without your regular routine. Perhaps you go to a regular exercise class or schedule exercise on a near daily basis. You may be a competitive athlete, or perhaps you may compete in more than one sport.

Assessing Your Needs and Abilities

Looking at these three categories of fitness, you might think you fit neatly into one of them. However, you should only use the fitness level category as a starting point.

Professional Evaluation

Some women prefer to have a professional evaluation of their fitness level. This can be done in most major fitness centers, including some hospital gyms. If you are having trouble finding someone to perform this assessment, you might try a professional association that trains fitness instructors or personal trainers. Fitness evaluation is a basic skill of personal trainers and fitness instructors.

A few practitioners might require a professional evaluation before giving you the go-ahead to exercise. If your doctor or midwife requests one from you, ask if he or she has a recommendation for where to have your fitness levels tested. In most cases, you will be able to use self-evaluation to figure out where to begin your exercise routine.

Self-Evaluation

Begin your self-evaluation by asking yourself the following questions about your body, your pregnancy, and exercise:

- What injuries have you experienced in the past (including broken bones, accidents, falls, previous surgeries, or other problems)?
- Do you have old injuries that still require nurturing? If so, can you find ways to alter different exercises to accommodate this injury?
- What medical conditions, if any, did you have before your pregnancy (e.g., chronic conditions including high blood pressure, heart disease, diabetes, arthritis, etc.)? Are they under control now? Do you have any specific concerns about these conditions?
- Are you suffering from current pregnancy discomforts (e.g., swelling, nausea, backache, etc.)?
- Have you developed potential complications during pregnancy, like gestational diabetes, anemia, or pregnancy induced hypertension (PIH)? If so, how can you still fit in exercise? Will there be restrictions on which exercises you are able to complete?

Regular Consultation with Your Practitioner

You will be meeting with your practitioner often throughout pregnancy. Initially, your visits will be monthly, and then later they will become weekly, so there will be an opportunity for constant re-evaluation during pregnancy. Your practitioner can help guide you as you grow in your pregnant body and continue to exercise.

fit as a fiddle

Chapter 10

Stress Busters

As you learn to exercise your body, so you must learn to exercise your mind. Relaxation can be done by anyone, in any location. The benefits are amazing for the body and soul. Pregnancy is a very beneficial time to learn the techniques of relaxation to aid you throughout life.

Stress and Pregnancy

Stress is something that we have come to expect as a society. Everywhere you go people are rushing. We learn vocabulary words like multitasking and pressure headaches. We learn that time is of the essence. Time is money. Stress is no longer a "four-letter word," but a societal ideal to which we are slaves.

During pregnancy the stresses of the physical body are many. You may spend a lot of time, effort, and even money to rid yourself of the physical problems that can be associated with pregnancy. When you add the mental and emotional stress of pregnancy to the physical stresses, the physical and nonphysical tension can be intense. There are many signs that scream to you that your body is under stress:

- Headaches
- Fatigue
- Tightness in your body
- Blood pressure problems
- Clenching teeth
- Heartburn and other intestinal restlessness disorders
- Insomnia
- Weight loss or gain

Why Stress Relief Is Important

No matter how you slice it, stress does not paint a pretty picture for your body. The tolls of stress on the nonpregnant body are slightly easier to recover from. However, during pregnancy the added toll of stress to your already taxed system has the potential to cause problems with the pregnancy in extreme situations.

·········· **need to know** ··························

Increased levels of stress can also affect how you absorb your nutrients, and prevent or restrict blood flow through the placenta to your baby, causing fetal growth restriction.

Stress can affect how you bond prenatally with your baby. Untreated stress can make life changes more difficult, particularly those you are trying to change for the benefit of your baby, for example, quitting smoking or changing eating habits.

Even if your stress levels have not reached the extremes required to harm the pregnancy, the stress you experience can make pregnancy more difficult for you. This has led to a huge increase in stress relief products and programs.

Stress relief happens in a variety of ways. From the physical to the mental, it is important to our well-being. One of the easiest ways to reduce stress is through relaxation. There are several types of relaxation and each one plays a part in your total body makeup. To neglect a component of this organization is to neglect your body. The three forms of relaxation are mental, emotional, and physical.

Mental Relaxation

Mental relaxation is probably the most widely talked about form of relaxation. If you are taking childbirth classes, you may have gone into great detail on this form of relaxation. Basically, the definition of mental relaxation is to be able to clear your mind of intrusive thoughts during certain periods.

The benefits of being able mentally to let go of ideas and extraneous thoughts is fairly obvious. You can clear your mind to deal with whatever it is you are currently doing. This type of relaxation is a focal point, to borrow a term from Lamaze, for many programs, including childbirth classes.

There are many ways to deal with mental stress. The one that is most available to you will probably be education. While education may sound like a simple answer to a complex problem, it is very often all you will need to help address the issues you are facing mentally in pregnancy.

If you are a fact- or detail-oriented person, this may not be a difficult task for you. Perhaps you've signed up for every class your birthing place offers. Maybe you've read some books on the topic. Chances are you've sought out some form of information about pregnancy, labor, and parenting to help you cope with the mental stresses of the unknowns. Even if this is not your first pregnancy, the issues of adding an additional person to your family or the stresses of things you would like to change from your first pregnancy can be many.

Emotional Relaxation

Emotional relaxation is the second hardest form of relaxation to learn. As the term implies, it has to do with dealing with the emotional issues that are affecting your life. During pregnancy, the emotional issues are many. Add hormones to the mix and you've got an interesting pot of feelings to deal with. You might be dealing with issues of becoming a parent for the first time. This leaves you revisiting issues of your childhood, both positive and negative. You may start to look at other parents you know and wonder what type of parents you and your partner will be.

Physical Relaxation

Contrary to popular belief, physical relaxation is much easier to achieve than mental or emotional relaxation. Your body's reaction to physical issues can be dealt with in a much clearer and more precise manner. The tools you have available to you are numerous and should be used as often as you wish. Some examples of these tools include:

- Massage
- Acupuncture
- Aromatherapy
- Hydrotherapy
- Music

Many of these tools can be used in conjunction with one another. For example, during a massage you may use some scented oils to aid in your relaxation or perhaps you listen to the radio while you take a bath. Sometimes you use these tools without being aware of their use or that you are deriving benefits from them. Think of how you feel when one of your favorite songs comes on the radio. First, you might tap your toes or fingers, but before you know it you are singing along, even when it is not necessarily appropriate. This is your body responding positively to something you enjoy.

.... **pregnancy treat** ....

Your body responds with the production of endorphins, hormones that make you naturally feel pleasant and relaxed.

While these tools are available for your use, even during pregnancy, they are not necessary for physical relaxation. They should be looked at merely as aids in the relaxation process. You will learn some physical relaxation techniques later in the chapter, such as the tense-release exercises, that use only your own body versus choosing to incorporate your partner into your physical relaxation for assistance. Do whatever makes you feel comfortable. Exercise is one of the best ways to deal with the physical stresses of life.

Exercise and Stress Relief

Exercise has always been a great way to deal with stress. Not only are there the obvious physical benefits of exercise, but now we are starting to recognize the stress-relieving benefits as well. In fact, many health-care providers recommend exercise as the number-one method of stress relief.

Distraction Techniques

Distraction techniques do just what they promise—they distract you. The best pregnancy based example I can offer is patterned paced breathing for labor. By focusing on your breathing rather than contractions, you use your mind to focus on something other than the contractions and discomfort. When practiced diligently it works really well, but practice is the key. This type of relaxation is beneficial for you if you harbor fear or tension related to a process or if escape is a common coping technique for you in life, in general.

The breath focusing of patterned paced breathing is used in many forms. One technique is to focus on the in and out breaths as you breathe. You can do this easily by slowly counting to ten and breathing in through your mouth. Hold that breath for a few comfortable seconds and then release your breath to the count of ten through your nose. If you find that ten seconds is too long, or too short, feel free to alter this number to whatever works well for you. Some also find that they prefer mouth breathing to nose breathing, so use whatever method of breathing feels natural to you.

This is but one example of a distraction technique. There are many others that you can use to help aid in relaxation throughout life. Some require even less thought than breathing, like listening to music, or watching movies or television. Many times you become so familiar with whatever method you choose that when a stressful situation comes up you do not even realize that you have reverted to doing your distraction technique.

Internal Focus Techniques

Through internal focus, you can directly address concerns about your body by using your mind. The benefit of using an internal focus can be that you are able to focus directly on your situation. Many of these techniques are used in childbirth classes and include focusing on the thoughts associated with the processes you are going through. These techniques work really well for you if you are fact-focused and interested in learning everything you can. This can also help alleviate fears associated with certain processes.

Mental Imagery

Mental imagery is simply defined as the ability to "see" images or scenes. This practice is used as a coping mechanism that can either be distracting or an internal focus. These techniques are used by many athletes before competition to improve performance.

Common types of mental images used in birth are those that are open and flowing. You can use waves to imagine a contraction pattern. You might use the image of a flower opening, like a rose bud, to imagine what your cervix is doing during labor.

The Perfect Memory

Many people choose to use a time and place that they have actually experienced to aid them in their relaxation. Using this mental imagery is very beneficial. You can choose any time or place that provides you with a positive memory. Be sure to recall as many physical and emotional details as possible. Things to remember include what you were wearing, who you were with, who said what, what smells were around you, what time of day or year it was. Was it a special occasion? You can choose a variety of situations, like your most romantic memory, a great vacation, a family getaway, and so forth. Is your memory perhaps merely a favorite place? A childhood safe haven or vacation home often works well. The key is to choose something or someplace that makes you feel good and safe.

The Birth Exercise

Using mental imagery to conjure up the birth of your baby can be a valuable tool. Simply use techniques to picture what you would like to happen during this special time. You might incorporate some of the facts you've learned about your body and childbirth in general to help you imagine your baby's birth.

·········· **pregnancy treat** ··········

This mental rehearsing is a great way to prepare yourself for the experience, even though it is not likely to go exactly as you have imagined it. It will also help reduce your prenatal anxiety and the stresses you feel once labor has begun.

To do this exercise, get in a relaxing position and set the mood with music and lighting if desired. Start with how you imagine your labor beginning and slowly proceed through the birth as you see it happening. If there is something or someplace where you get "stuck" and can't envision, do not panic, move on. It will come. You can end at any point. Some end their imaginings with the birth of the baby, so you might choose to end there or a bit further postpartum.

You can also do this with your husband or partner. Allow him or her to tell you the story of the birth while you focus on the physical relaxation. This can help you work through differences the two of you have in philosophy or experience. Don't hesitate to say how you imagine it all working out.

Tense-Release Exercises

Tense-release exercises are the most basic form of physical relaxation. You probably use these techniques without even realizing that you are doing them. Clenching your fists and relaxing them, for example, is something many of us do if we're angry. Perhaps when you feel a tension headache coming on, you might scrunch your neck up and then extend it a bit. These are all tense-release exercises. You can use the tense-release technique consciously to help alleviate tension in muscles throughout your pregnancy.

·········· **pregnancy treat** ··········

One of the great things about tense-release exercises is that they can be done in nearly any situation. These can even be done if you experience complications.

To do a formal tense-release exercise, assume a comfortable position; this can be sitting or lying down. You can set the mood with music or dimmed lighting if you desire. Start at the top of your body—your head. Scrunch your forehead up as tightly as you can. Hold the tension for up to five seconds. Then, deliberately release the tension from your forehead. Experience the difference between the tension previously felt and the current state of relaxation. Invite your partner or coach to experience your tension and relaxation both visually and by the use of touch. This will help him or her guide you in labor.

Next, go lower and scrunch your face and ears. Hold for five seconds and release. Now tighten your neck so that your ears rest on your shoulders. Hold this for an additional five seconds and again release. Tighten your back, holding for five seconds and releasing. Now do the same with your arms and hands, holding the tension for five seconds and releasing the tension. Next scrunch your buttocks and hips; hold for five and release. Proceed to do the same with your thighs, and then your lower legs and feet.

For an added "workout," have your partner massage you to help you learn to release the tension. To do this, simply have your partner begin to massage the tensed area three to four seconds into the holding phase of the tension.

Touch Therapy and Massage

Touch is usually a very positive thing for most people, so when you add to that the benefits of touch on healing and physical and emotional well-being, we know that the benefits are many. Massage is commonly used in athletics as a form of physical therapy, but it can also be used to relax and ease the mental and physical stressors of pregnancy. The physical benefits of massage on pregnancy are numerous.

Massage can also help increase and improve your circulation, a must when your pregnant body is dealing with an ever-expanding blood volume. It can also help with swelling issues and problems related to stress, such as insomnia and blood pressure concerns.

Massage can be done at nearly any point in pregnancy. Some massage practitioners will schedule massages in blocks of time from fifteen to seventy-five minutes depending on your personal needs. There is no one right answer for how often you can or should have a massage.

Finding a Massage Practitioner

There are many organizations that certify or train massage therapy practitioners. Some actually offer certifications in pregnancy and the childbearing year. You should always interview the person you are working with, even if it is someone you have been seeing for years, about their knowledge of pregnancy and its related issues. Your massage therapist should be forthcoming about his or her training. Some may even request a specific release from your doctor or midwife to allow you to continue receiving massages throughout pregnancy. Some practitioners of massage will not perform massages on women who are less than twelve weeks' gestation. While massage has never been implicated in early miscarriage, it is important to talk to your doctor or midwife and your massage therapist about concerns related to your physical well-being in pregnancy.

Your Massage Experience

If you have never had a massage before, you might be wondering what actually happens during a massage. Part of what happens will depend on the type and length of massage, as well as your practitioner and your comfort levels. Generally speaking, massage is performed with you lying down on a special table, with a section cut out for your expanding abdomen, or with your body propped on pillow bolsters to prevent you from lying on your back. The room usually has dimmed lighting to promote relaxation.

.... **need to know** ....

Many therapists have you remove your clothing completely or down to the underwear, no bra. That said, there is a sheet and/or blanket used to cover you during the entire massage.

Some forms of massage are done over the blanket to ensure your privacy, while still providing you with the best massage physically. Removing clothing is obviously not acceptable for all, and again is something you need to discuss with the practitioner.

Partner Massage

Professional massage, while nice, is not for everyone. You may, therefore, choose to supplement visits with your massage therapist with massages from your partner, or even a good friend.

Suggest to your partner that you practice some of the relaxation techniques you have learned prior to bed each night. This has the added benefits of relaxing you mentally and physically and can help you sleep more soundly.

Do not be fearful of how to massage someone. The techniques are easy to learn. Many childbirth classes incorporate massage into their class schedules because the benefit is so great. If you haven't yet signed up for a class, just tell your partner what feels good or what is hurting. Massage tends to be a pretty instinctual experience. If the massage you receive isn't exactly what you need, offer to massage your partner the way you'd like to be massaged. This usually gets the message across very efficiently.

As you see, relaxation is a key to understanding the body's processes throughout life and particularly during pregnancy. As stress can have a negative impact on your physical, mental, and emotional well-being, you need to be aware of the tension that can gather in your body. Using the tools discussed in this chapter, you can reduce the negative effects of stress and tension on your mind and body. This will also help prepare you for the roller coaster of parenting.

stress busters

Chapter 11

Career Concerns

*W*orried about keeping up on the job during your pregnancy? Recognize your value, not just as an employee but also as a woman. Don't let anyone make you feel guilty about being pregnant. Know your rights, stick to your guns, and realize you don't have to settle for the status quo when it comes to the workplace.

Your Rights

Unfortunately, it's sometimes easier to change the legal employment landscape than alter prevalent workplace attitudes and prejudices. Too frequently, pregnancy is construed as a personal indication that you have no want or need for professional fulfillment.

Even if you do consider work nothing more than a way to pay the bills, your rights are still important. Intolerant and illegal attitudes toward pregnancy can result in financial loss as career advancement screeches to a halt, you get the minimum salary bump at your annual review, and bigger and better job offers dry up. Fortunately, federal and state statutes are in place to try to minimize the chance that you will be professionally or economically punished for your choice to become a mother.

The Pregnancy Discrimination Act

The Pregnancy Discrimination Act is a 1978 amendment to Title VII of the Civil Rights Act of 1964. The act requires that your employer provide you with the same rights, accommodations, and benefits as other employees who are on temporary disability due to illness or injury. It also dictates that your employer must allow you to work as long as you are physically able to do your job. The act only applies to businesses with more than fifteen employees, and if your employer does not provide disability benefits to injured or ill employees, your comparable benefits will be just that—nothing. If you're searching for a new position while pregnant, the Pregnancy Discrimination Act protects you from prejudice on the basis of your pregnancy.

···················· **need to know** ····························

It's illegal for a potential employer to ask if you're pregnant or not in the interview, and you certainly aren't required to volunteer the information.

If the job is offered to you, it is probably in your best interest to mention your pregnancy during final negotiations. You want to start your working relationship off on the right foot and address any concerns your prospective employer has up front.

The Family and Medical Leave Act (FMLA)

If you or your spouse work for a public agency, a private or public elementary or secondary school, or a company with more than fifty employees for a period of at least a year, you have coverage under the Family Medical Leave Act (FMLA).

The FMLA also enables you to take unpaid time off if you experience health problems during pregnancy and your employer does not provide disability or sick day benefits. The same goes for extended time off you might require to care for your child should she have any health problems at birth. Again, the total time off provided for under the FMLA is not to exceed a total of twelve weeks in twelve months.

State Law

Depending on where you live, your state may mandate certain employee rights related to pregnancy and maternity benefits under Worker's Compensation laws. Check with the labor department or other applicable organization in your state to find out more.

Occupational Hazards

Depending on your position and work environment, you may have to alter your duties temporarily, or request a change in location or accommodations. If your job involves any of the following elements, talk with your human resources department about your options:

Weight lifting. Lifting heavy packages, boxes, or other items is not recommended in pregnancy, especially past twenty weeks (e.g., shipping and receiving clerks, warehouse work).

Secondhand smoke. Women who work in the hospitality industry (e.g., bartenders, waitresses) may expose their fetus to toxins in secondhand smoke. Thankfully, more states are banning smoking in all public places, including restaurants and bars.

High heat. Excessive temperatures can be harmful to fetal development, particularly in the first trimester (e.g., summer construction, factory environment).

Teratogen exposure. Jobs that involve working with certain chemicals and hazardous substances (e.g., welders and lead exposure) are linked to birth defects.

continued

career concerns

Standing and repetitive movement. Line work or other jobs that keep you on your feet all day (e.g., factory jobs, assembly work, piece work) can exacerbate circulatory problems.

Ionizing radiation exposure. Pregnant pilots and flight crew may be exposed to excessive ionizing radiation, another known teratogen. Radiographic imaging technicians that work with X rays, CT scanning equipment, and nuclear medicine are also at risk.

Breaking the News

In an ideal world, the news of your impending motherhood would be greeted with congratulations and reassurance at the office. Instead, reality may find you strategizing against a negative employer reaction and determining the right time to drop the pregnancy bombshell. That pregnancy should be considered a handicap to be overcome rather than the positive, life-affirming force it is remains a glaring reminder of how far women still have to go to achieve equality in the workplace.

When you do inform your employer, make sure that they hear it from you first. Accompany the news with your tentative schedule for maternity leave so your manager can plan accordingly. Offering suggestions you have for a replacement in your absence or ways to temporarily reassign workload will reflect well on you and your perceived commitment to your employer.

Avoiding the "Mommy Track" Trap

Once you share your news, you may suddenly find yourself on a slow road to nowhere at work—last in the information loop and out of the running for promotions and job advancements you were previously an easy pick for. Goodbye fast track and hello mommy track?

Is it unavoidable? Not necessarily. Employers who realize that a happy employee is more likely to be a productive employee won't punish you for pursuing a personal life. And if you continue to perform well and make it clear to your supervisors and management that you'd like to have a career path with the company rather than just a job, you're more likely to avoid the so-called mommy track. Still, whether the mommy track exists in your organization or not depends on the corporate culture and the attitudes of upper management. Do they support family-friendly policies? Do they lead by example and use benefits like paternity leave themselves? And are efforts made to institute initiatives that benefit employees across the board, from the security staff to the CEO?

Defining Personal and Professional Goals

What do you want out of life, both personally and professionally, now that your family is changing? If this is your first child, it can be hard to fully assess the new direction you're taking. But there are probably some basic decisions you can make with a degree of certainty. For example, late shifts and double-overtime may be out of the picture for you now. You may also have career goals that you'd like to keep on target. Should they be mutually exclusive of motherhood? No. May they be, depending on where you work? Yes. If you wanted to move into a supervisory position at your next review, but see your company promoting those who work excessive overtime, you have choices to make. Such is the delicate balance of motherhood.

Fortunately, you always have the option to look for a workplace that is more in harmony with your personal and professional goals—or to take your own path, whatever it may be.

Realize Your Value

Think of full-time motherhood as another job offer on the table for your employer to stack up to.

·········· **need to know** ··························

Your company may be willing to sweeten the pot with flex-time, telecommuting, or other family-friendly working arrangements to keep you happy.

Remember, in most cases they have poured a significant amount of money and resources into your training. The loss of that investment, plus the cost of hiring and training a new employee, is a big financial incentive for keeping you on board. Don't be afraid to rock the boat. Realize your value and use it as a bargaining chip.

Negotiate Toward Your Goal

Think about using your maternity leave as a launchpad for alternate working arrangements. For example, if you would like more than the six weeks of paid leave your company offers and would ultimately like some flexibility in your schedule, suggest a work arrangement like telecommuting for the six weeks following paid leave. If you're covered by the FMLA, your employer must give you twelve weeks off without pay to care for your newborn if you request it. By offering an alternative to your complete absence, you appear flexible and dedicated, and your employer certainly has nothing to lose by trying it. Even if you aren't prepared to take six weeks off unpaid should your employer turn you down, it's well worth the gamble to suggest the idea. You can always scale back your plans if your request isn't granted. And if it is accepted and works out well, you will have proven yourself for a more permanent arrangement down the road.

Practical Matters

No matter what your job, staying comfortable, relatively stress-free, and economically secure during your pregnancy is essential.

Staying Comfortable

Women who work on their feet should make a habit of changing positions often and moving when possible. Wear comfortable shoes and consider support stockings. For jobs that require a lot of sit-down time, make sure you have an ergonomically appropriate chair that promotes good posture.

career concerns

If you work a desk job, look for opportunities to get up and about. Take a walk to speak with a coworker instead of picking up the phone or hand-deliver a memo instead of using interoffice e-mail.

·   need to know   ·

A lumbar support pad may also help ease pregnancy-related lower back pain, and you can put up your feet under your desk on a small stool or even a stack of phonebooks.

Scheduling Doctor Visits

Hopefully, your employer recognizes that good prenatal care translates to a healthier, more productive employee and in the long run, less time spent out of the office to care for sick kids. However, if you do face resistance in taking time off for doctor's visits, remember that prenatal care is considered necessary medical care and is covered under the FMLA. If all else fails, you can invoke your legal rights. In the meantime, find out if your provider has evening, weekend, or early morning appointments that might fit around your workday. If you must go during office hours and your supervisor isn't pleased, offer her the alternative option of taking the entire day of your appointment off as vacation or unpaid leave instead. Perhaps she'll look at your short absence in a new light. If you're getting static for meeting basic prenatal care requirements now, just think what it will be like when you need time off to care for a sick child or keep a

the "i have a life" pregnancy guide

well-baby appointment. File a "family unfriendly" mental note for follow up postpregnancy.

If too many red flags are raised during your pregnancy, once you reach maternity leave it may be time to look for a company that realizes the value of both personal and professional fulfillment in their employees.

Controlling Stress

The workplace can be a stress hotbed. Deadlines, personality conflicts, difficult clients, quotas, overtime, and more make for a pressure cooker that's not good for you or baby. Try to maintain some perspective and peace of mind by realizing that petty office politics mean little in comparison to the health and well-being of your child.

Maternity Leave

Your bonding time with baby should be free of workplace concerns. If you plan appropriately for your departure and absence as early as possible, you'll get more out of your time off. It's a good idea to put all maternity leave plans in writing for your supervisor and appropriate managers, and to make an extra copy for placement in your personnel file.

Planning Ahead for Leave

Lay the groundwork for your maternity leave so there won't be too many questions or crises in your absence. If appropriate for your position, delegate some tasks to coworkers and arrange coverage by others. Find out if your supervisor plans on hiring temporary help to fill in during your absence, and work on training materials and checklists so you won't face a mess upon your return to the office. Check and double-check that all appropriate benefits paperwork has been filled out, signed off, and sent in well in advance of your planned departure. Maternity leave should be a low-stress time, not one that requires twice weekly contact with human resources to find out the status of your disability claim.

How Many Weeks?

So just how much, or how little, maternity leave should you take? Certainly the benefits your company provides will play a major factor in your decision. If you have quite a bit of seniority you may be able to swing an even longer leave by tapping into accrued vacation time. Other factors to consider include:

Money. How much time off can you afford if your maternity benefits are minimal or nonexistent? Don't forget to factor any money you'll be saving (i.e., dry cleaning bills, lunches out, transportation expenses) into your equation.

Management. Even though you may be legally within your rights, in some organizations an extended maternity leave may be frowned upon by those above you. Consider what management might think, and more importantly, what kind of priority you should place on their disapproval.

Morale. Are your coworkers and/or subordinates happy and motivated, or disillusioned and bitter? Employees that work as a team and feel invested in their workplace are more likely to rise to the challenge in your absence.

Malleability. Does it have to be all or nothing? Think about offering some creative proposals for extending your leave, such as a reduced part-time schedule or telecommuting.

Evaluating your leave options will reveal your company's attitudes toward personal employee fulfillment. Once you've gotten past maternity leave it may be time to consider your options.

Back to Work

After you actually deliver your child, the toughest job you'll have is that first day back to work. You'll worry about whether his caregiver will be able to tell his hungry cry from his tired cry, if he's getting the attention he thrives on, and of course if he misses you. Try to focus on the benefits of the situation—the increased value of the time you do have together, his broadening horizons as he interacts with new children and adults, and the financial security your family is gaining.

Easing the Transition

No matter how you slice it, it's hard being away from your baby. If you can, start back on half days to ease into the separation. Drop in at day care during your lunch hour if it's logistically possible. Above all, make the most of the time you do have together by making home a work-free zone.

Striking a Balance

In your premommy life, you may have set up certain expectations you find yourself hard pressed to live up to now. It's time to define appropriate work limits, even if it means pulling in old boundaries. Coworkers and clients who felt free to contact you before via pagers, wireless phones, or what have you, day or night, now need to be gently guided to keeping it to the office or at the least evaluating the urgency of their issues before picking up the phone. Getting some control back may be as simple as gradually ridding yourself of all the extra gadgetry that makes you painfully accessible and weaning your colleagues to voicemail or e-mail only access. Women who work nontraditional schedules may have special needs for achieving balance. Evening "day care" can be tough to find without friends or relatives in the area, and scheduling that changes on a weekly basis can make child care even more difficult to plan on. Talk to your supervisor candidly about your needs and see if a shift change or a more permanent schedule can be arranged.

Chapter 12

Labor Roadmap: Your Birth Plan

You've picked a provider, scouted out a birthplace, and surrounded yourself with the perfect support team. Don't forget your birth plan—your script for staging the best birth experience possible. Planning ahead and getting your expectations down on paper will not only help you get organized, it will give you a chance to discuss your wishes with your provider in advance and avoid unpleasant surprises on the big day.

Why Have a Birth Plan?

Like everything in life, labor and birth are unpredictable. No two occasions are alike, even with the same woman. So why even develop a birth plan? First of all, putting your expectations and wishes on paper gets everyone on your birth team, from your provider to any friends and family who may be present, on the same page.

Also, the very process of creating your birth plan enables you and your partner to discover what you want to get out of your birth experience, to prioritize your needs and wishes, and to resolve any potential disagreements now rather than during labor. Finally, a birth plan allows you to express your wishes about interventions (such as use of forceps, anesthesia and analgesia use, or episiotomy) should the issue arise. Making informed decisions ahead of time can save you the stress of making difficult choices during the birth.

.... **need to know** ....

When your birth plan is finalized, ask your provider to place a copy of it both in your chart and hospital record. Any support people who will be attending the birth should also be given a copy to familiarize themselves with.

In simplest form, your birth plan is an outline of what you and your partner want, and don't want, during labor and birth. To be most effective, a birth plan should be brief; anything over five pages is probably too much. It should use cooperative language ("would like" and "prefer" rather than "must have" and "demand") and leave room for alternatives in case complications arise.

Staging Your Birth

Your comfort level and peace of mind on the big birth day will have a direct impact on how your labor progresses. Working out what may seem like minor details now and clearing possible points of contention with your provider will make the birth itself that much easier and anxiety-free.

Atmosphere

So what's the ambiance of your chosen birthplace? Is it a four-poster bed and sunshine through cheery floral curtains, or white tile and chrome with an antiseptic scent?

Your birth plan can include a list of items from home to bring to the hospital. And remember those hospital-issue foam slippers are no replacement for your own fuzzy favorites.

Music is also a great tool for relaxation, lifting your mood, providing focus, and getting the adrenaline going when it's time to push. Stick with a play list you can control—you don't want to be perpetually dialing past farm reports to get in a station or stuck in a place with bad reception. Creating your own CD or tape with a varied repertoire is a good idea. For example, include selections of classical music to relax you, along with something more up-tempo to motivate you in active labor.

If you want to listen to music during labor and delivery, make sure your birth facility allows the use of a portable stereo, and do keep in mind

labor roadmap: your birth plan

that depending on where your birth is planned, there may be other women laboring who would appreciate some volume control. Worse case scenario, you have to wear headphones, so it's a good idea to prepare for this by having a pair available. You may want to invest in an extra-long cord as well.

The lighting can also make a big difference in your mood and comfort. The harsh fluorescent fixtures that are common in many hospitals may not create a very restful environment.

Your birth plan can include a request that the lights be dimmed and the curtains drawn if lower light helps relax you during labor and birth. A darkened environment might ease her transition into this new world as well.

Cast and Crew

You've already made decisions about the health-care professional who will be attending your birth. You've also decided on a primary support person, or two, to have on your team. Depending on your personal situation and preferences, these may be the only attendees you will have onboard for this performance. If your young children are going to be present at the birth of their sibling, be sure to arrange to have a caregiver there to provide supervision and support, even if you're giving birth at home. You and your partner will have your hands full with other things.

However, you may have a bigger cast in mind. Are you thinking about having your children participate in the birth in some capacity? Do you want family and close friends present at the birth, or waiting in the wings nearby? Your birth plan should spell out your expectations in this respect.

Props

Beyond comfort objects to "warm up" your labor and birth room, what kind of items do you want to have access to for pain relief and/or labor assistance? Some items may be supplied by your birth place, while others may have to be brought in. Objects to consider include these:

Shower or whirlpool. Most birth centers and many hospitals now offer a whirlpool tub and/or shower to ease labor pain.

A birth ball. Sitting and/or rocking on this large inflatable rubber ball encourages perineal relaxation and pelvic mobility. Some women also lean against the birth ball on hands and knees to ease back labor pain.

Birthing stool. A birth stool is a seatless or partial-seat stool that allows a woman to deliver in a natural squatting position while providing support.

Massage devices. Massage from a partner or doula during labor can be a great relaxation technique. There are dozens of devices available on the market, but a small rolling pin or a sock containing tennis balls can sometimes fit the bill quite nicely.

A cooler. A small cooler can come in handy for cold compresses, light snacks, and drinks.

Some hospitals may try to limit you to ice chips and other fluid nourishments. While a meatball sandwich is probably not the best choice during active labor, there's nothing wrong with something light to keep your strength and energy up if you are having a normal, low-risk birth.

Check with your facility for information on access to any equipment you might need. Your midwife and/or doula may also have some of this equipment on hand to provide as part of her services. If it isn't available and you want it, buy or rent it early so you can bring it with you on the big day.

Head Shots

Like every modern parent, you probably are planning to capture a portion of the big event for posterity. Including your photographic expectations in your birth plan helps you ensure that they pass muster with your birth facility and gives you a checklist when it comes time to pack. It's possible you don't want your partner snapping pictures of every contraction instead of attending to your needs. Written requests stating that photos should only be taken during certain stages of labor and birth, or only when you ask for them, can prevent your overzealous shutterbug from getting carried away.

While birthing centers are usually amenable to any requests you have regarding photographing and recording the birth, getting the pictures you want may be a bit trickier if you're planning a hospital birth. There may be rules against filming of the actual birth itself or regulations forbidding the use of any special equipment, such as a tripod, that might get in the way. With today's tiny digital recorders, some of these fears of bulky equipment getting in the way and wires to trip over may be unwarranted. Talk to your hospital and provider about these issues so you can know what to expect.

Planning with Your Provider

Reviewing your birth plan with your provider well in advance of your due date is essential. If there are any aspects of the plan your provider disagrees with or will potentially refuse to comply with, you want to know early rather than being faced with an unpleasant surprise while in labor.

·························· **need to know** ··························

Many physicians and midwives will schedule a separate office visit for the primary purpose of going over your birth plan. If your provider doesn't suggest one, take it upon yourself to ask for a dedicated appointment to review your needs and wishes.

Ask your provider and hospital or birth center about their fetal monitoring policy. Walking in labor can ease discomfort and speed progress for many women, but being tethered to a monitor can prevent you from moving through contractions. With a low-risk birth, intermittent (that is, occasional) monitoring should not be a problem in most facilities.

Consider the version of the birth plan you take in to your provider to be a first draft, open to revision. Some practitioners may get defensive about the idea of a birth plan, believing that it conveys a lack of trust in their clinical abilities. Others may be concerned that if complications arise and the birth goes off-course from the plan, they may have a disappointed patient on their hands. And some physicians are simply grounded in the notion that their job is to "deliver" the baby rather than let the patient give birth and own the birth experience.

An open and honest approach can help dissuade any negative feelings about the birth plan. Being receptive to suggestions and communicative, rather than defensive, can do a lot toward lowering your provider's guard and getting him or her to work effectively on your plan.

Getting Everyone on the Same Page

So how do you make sure that your birth plan both reflects your needs and will be accepted (and more importantly, followed appropriately) by your provider? First, while you may have firmly grounded expectations of your birth, be willing to listen to the proposals and issues your provider may have and to work together toward a resolution.

Here are some other tips for getting the most out of your plan:

- Make requests, not demands. Keep the language cooperative and communicative so your provider doesn't feel intimidated by the tone.
- Get to the point. Think brevity and bullet points. The medical staff that attends your birth needs to be able to see your wishes clearly and quickly, especially if time is of the essence.
- Short and sweet. Don't present your provider with the Encyclopedia Britannica. You don't need to choreograph every contraction.

- Convey trust. Let your midwife or physician know that you trust her to follow the spirit of your birth plan.
- Offer alternatives. Be sure to outline your wishes regarding interventions in case complications arise.

Being Prepared: Interventions

Even the best-laid birth plans can go awry. One of the most important elements of a birth plan is a section on provisions for the unexpected. Some women may feel that they "failed" at birth when things don't end up exactly as planned. By building alternative scenarios into your birth plan, you can lessen any later disappointments.

Look at possible worst-case scenarios. Outline your preferences should interventions have to happen, and state your wishes regarding steps to be taken to prevent interventions. For example, you may want to ask for a trial of perineal massage and compresses if your perineum isn't stretching adequately to allow for baby's exit before allowing an episiotomy to occur.

Your pain-management preferences will be a big part of your birth plan. If you take prepared childbirth classes, you'll learn about some options there, and your provider can also outline options for you.

It's also a good idea to include a section about your preferences regarding cesarean birth, even if yours is a normal low-risk pregnancy and you plan on delivering vaginally. Cover such issues as type of anesthesia, presence of your coach, being able to view the birth, and who will hold and be with the baby first. You will probably never need such provisions, but if you do, it will be one less thing to worry about when the time comes.

need to know

If you're interested in natural birth, a midwife or doula may be a better source of information than a physician, as her experience in nonmedicated births tends to be broader.

Try not to be so restrictive in your language that your provider feels like her hands are tied in your care. And remember that as labor progresses, it's possible that you may want to make some adjustments to the birth plan as well. You may plan on an epidural and then decide during labor that you don't need it. Or you may decide on having a natural childbirth and in the end decide that some pharmaceutical pain relief is the right thing for you. As long as you have an active and self-determined part in any alterations to the plan, last-minute changes are normal and acceptable.

If you're having a planned cesarean section for whatever reason, it's likely that the hospital will have specific rules and regulations regarding operative procedure. However, there are certain things you can and should have a say in that a birth plan can help pin down.

Talk to your doctor about what may be flexible (such as seeing the birth in a well-placed mirror or having your significant other cut the cord) and what is nonnegotiable (things like anesthesia or surgical prep).

The Perfect Debut

Is there any moment more powerful than your first face-to-face with your newborn? By the time this moment comes, you will have spent nearly ten months dreaming about it, possibly years more if pregnancy was difficult to achieve. Of course you want it to be just right, so take the time to think about and include your preferences in your birth plan.

> ### pregnancy treat
>
> Barring any complications, birthing centers typically let you and your family spend as much time cuddling and bonding with the new baby as you'd like before doing any routine fingerprinting or testing.

As your first official parental duty in a birthing center, you and your partner help and hold baby during the weigh-in, measurement, and after-birth cleanup. There is no separation involved.

A hospital, on the other hand, may have certain protocols in place for newborn care, including immediate blood tests, eyedrops, heat lamps, and vitamin K injections. If you're planning a hospital birth, talk to your care provider and a hospital representative now to find out what the exact protocols are. A few questions to ask include these: Will you be allowed to hold your newborn skin-to-skin while the placenta is delivered and she is evaluated, or will you just get a peek and a promise of a swift return? Do you or your partner have the option to cut the cord, and must it be done immediately? If the baby requires medical attention at birth, will your partner be allowed to stay with her? It's a good idea to educate yourself on the issues surrounding newborn tests and procedures now so you can inquire about policy and state your wishes in your birth plan. Even if the protocol is very strict, at the very least you will know what to expect.

························· **need to know** ·························

Vitamin K assists in blood clotting and is usually formed in the intestinal tract, but newborns aren't able to produce it at birth.

In the early 1990s, several studies found an association between vitamin K at birth and childhood cancers; however, subsequent studies have found no link between the two. While vitamin K is usually given by injection shortly after birth, studies have also found that several oral doses of vitamin K are just as effective and possibly less traumatic for both you and your child.

Postpartum Preplanning

Your birth plan doesn't end with baby's entrance into the world. Adding a postpartum section to the birth plan can be a big help in getting you organized and keeping you and baby on a reasonable schedule once your new family is back at home. Following are some things you might want to include.

Maternity and paternity leave. If you and/or your partner are taking it, outline how much and when (for example, six weeks from the due date, twelve weeks after birth). Be sure to investigate your leave and insurance options.

Home support system. Will you have some live-in help for a few weeks, or are you flying solo?

Backup. Line up friends and neighbors who will make the occasional grocery store run, drop off a meal, or do other errands for you during those early days.

First meetings. Are close relatives or friends planning a visit after the birth, or are you keeping baby to yourself for a while?

Doctor's visits. Both you and baby will be visiting your respective doctors in the weeks following the birth. Put this on your birth plan now so you won't forget to schedule appointments when the time comes.

Remember, your birth plan can be a great tool in achieving the birth experience you and your partner want. Start early so you can make fully informed decisions and work with your provider to make the plan workable to everyone involved. The following birth plan checklist can help guide you through the process.

1. Where will the birth take place?
   - ○ Hospital
   - ○ Birthing center
   - ○ Home
   - ○ Other: _____

2. Who will be there for labor support?
   - ○ Husband or significant other
   - ○ Doula
   - ○ Friend
   - ○ Family member

3. Will any room modifications or equipment be required to increase your comfort mentally and physically?
   - ○ Objects from home (e.g., pictures, blanket, pillow)
   - ○ Lighting adjustments
   - ○ Music
   - ○ Video or photos of birth
   - ○ Other: _____

4. Any special requests for labor prep procedures?
   - ○ Forego enema
   - ○ Self-administer the enema
   - ○ Forego shaving
   - ○ Shave self
   - ○ Heparin lock instead of routine IV line
   - ○ Other: _____

5. Eating and drinking during labor?
   - ○ Want access to a light snack
   - ○ Want access to water, sports drink, or other appropriate beverage
   - ○ Want ice chips
   - ○ Other: _____

6. Do you want pain medication?
   - ○ Analgesic (e.g., Stadol, Demerol, Nubain)
   - ○ Epidural (if so, is timing an issue?)
   - ○ Other:

7. What nonpharmaceutical pain relief equipment might you want access to?
   - ○ Hydrotherapy (i.e., shower, whirlpool)
   - ○ Warm compresses
   - ○ Birth ball
   - ○ Other: _____

8. What interventions would you like to avoid unless deemed a medical necessity by your provider during labor? Specify your preferred alternatives.
   - ○ Episiotomy
   - ○ Forceps
   - ○ Internal fetal monitoring
   - ○ Pitocin (oxytocin)
   - ○ Other: _____

9. What would you like your first face-to-face with baby to be like?
   - ○ Hold off on all nonessential treatment, evaluation, and tests for a specified time
   - ○ If immediate tests and evaluation are necessary, you, your partner, or another support person will accompany baby
   - ○ Want to nurse immediately following birth
   - ○ Would like family members to meet baby immediately following birth
   - ○ Other: _____

10. If a cesarean birth is required, what is important to you and your partner?
    - ○ Type of anesthesia (e.g., general vs. spinal block)
    - ○ Having partner or another support person present
    - ○ Spending time with baby immediately following procedure
    - ○ Bonding with baby in the recovery room
    - ○ Type of postoperative pain relief and nursing considerations
    - ○ Other: _____

11. Do you have a preference for who cuts the cord and when the cut is performed?
    - ○ Mom   ○ Dad   ○ Provider
    - ○ Delay until cord stops pulsing
    - ○ Cord blood will be banked; cut per banking guidelines
    - ○ Cut at provider's discretion
    - ○ Other: _____

12. What kind of postpartum care will you and baby have at the hospital?
   - ○ Baby will room-in with mom
   - ○ Baby will sleep in the nursery at night
   - ○ Baby will breastfeed
   - ○ Baby will bottle feed
   - ○ Baby will not be fed any supplemental formula and/or glucose water unless medically indicated
   - ○ Baby will not be given a pacifier
   - ○ Other: _____
13. Considerations for after discharge:
   - ○ Support and short-term care for siblings
   - ○ Support if you've had a caesarean
   - ○ Maternity leave
   - ○ Other: _____

Chapter 13

The Birth Experience

Successful labor is a state of mind as much as it is a physical process. If you're anxious, scared, and stressed, your body will react with pain and resistance. Educating yourself about what to expect can really help you to achieve a positive, prepared state of mind. Once labor begins, being comfortable and in control of the labor process and working with your body instead of against it will make your birth experience more productive and enjoyable.

Emotional Barriers

"I don't know if I can do this" is a common refrain among first-time moms. Yes, childbirth is a challenge, but so is every other goal worth achieving in life. There will be pain, but it's positive pain—pain that is bringing your baby to the outside world. And don't forget that you have many tools at your disposal to work through that pain in your own way.

If you open your mind to your own potential and jettison any preconceived notions of birth, you'll realize you can do it—and do it quite well.

····················· **need to know** ·····················

It may sound clichéd, but the best way to ensure a good birth experience is
to believe in yourself and your abilities.

The Stages of Labor

Your baby may start preparing for birth before labor even begins by settling lower into your pelvis. Called "engagement," "lightening," or simply
"the baby dropping," this move downward places pressure on the cervix so
it can begin the task of effacement (thinning) and dilation (opening).

Not all women experience engagement prior to labor. Some babies,
particularly those born to second-time moms, may not move down into
the pelvic cavity until labor officially begins.

Labor itself is divided into three stages:

First stage: Lasts from early contractions until the cervix is ten
centimeters dilated.

Second stage: The pushing part; the actual delivery of your baby.

Third stage: Delivery of the placenta.

First Stage

Typically the longest phase of the labor process, the first phase consists
of three parts—early (latent) labor, active labor, and transition (descent)

labor. Your cervix may already begin to ripen well before early labor starts. When the first stage of labor begins, your uterine muscles will squeeze, causing you to feel contractions, and the cervix will dilate further—four to five centimeters during early labor. Contractions will be coming every fifteen to twenty minutes and should be between sixty and ninety seconds in duration. Once you've established that contractions are regular and real, contact your provider and other support people on your birth team to let them know the show has begun. If you have any bleeding or loss of fluid, or if you notice decreased fetal movement, contact your provider immediately to let him know what is going on. (According to the American College of Obstetricians and Gynecologists, normal fetal movement is ten fetal movements in a two-hour period.)

How will you know a "real" contraction when it comes? As any woman who has labored can tell you, you'll definitely know. In case you're still wary of missing the signal, a labor contraction is one that 1) causes discomfort that does not improve significantly when you change positions; 2) comes at roughly regular intervals; 3) increases in intensity as time passes; and 4) leads to a change in the cervix.

Your provider will instruct you on when to head for the hospital or birthing center or when she will come to you, should you be planning a home birth. Because early labor can be long, this probably won't be until you're approaching the active phase of the first stage of labor, where contractions are at regular three- to five-minute intervals and last approximately forty-five seconds each. The strong contractions of active labor will dilate your cervix to approximately eight centimeters when the transition phase starts.

Transition is perhaps the most difficult part of labor because your contractions are coming fast and furious, and you're faced with the overwhelming urge to push—but can't yet. As your cervix dilates those final two centimeters to a full ten, you'll feel intense pressure on your rectum from the baby's head, and severe back pain. It's normal to feel nauseous and have the chills or sweats. Breathing exercises can help you quell the urge to push until full dilation is achieved and stage two begins.

Second Stage

As the second stage starts, the baby descends into the vagina, or birth canal. Now you can finally push to help her along, and the elastic walls of your vagina will widen for her passage down the final five inches of the journey to the outside world. The gripping pain of contractions changes to a stinging or burning sensation as your perineum, the external tissue between the vaginal opening and anus, stretches to accommodate baby's emerging head and body. The burning sensation affects a circular area of the perineal tissues surrounding the vaginal opening. As the baby's head bulges out of your vaginal opening, your provider may ask you to stop pushing momentarily to prevent perineal tearing. This request may feel as futile as patching the Hoover Dam with a damp sponge, but panting can help you quash the urge to push until it's safe. Once you push the baby's head and shoulders out, the rest of her body will slide out easily by comparison.

If you aren't in the ideal pushing position to see your baby emerge, many hospitals and birthing centers offer mirrors to watch your baby as she enters the world. Ask when you tour the birth facility so you can know if you have the option.

Even if mirrors aren't available, you may be able to make arrangements to bring in a small mirror for your use.

Third Stage

Once you've been through stages one and two, the third stage of labor is a cakewalk. Your placenta must be delivered and examined to ensure that you haven't retained any pieces in your uterus. Your provider may suggest an injection of Pitocin to strengthen your contractions enough to deliver the placenta efficiently. Other providers may wait until after the placenta has been delivered to suggest giving Pitocin, in which case the goal is to increase uterine contractions in an attempt to decrease uterine bleeding.

Easing Baby's Passage

One of the most miraculous aspects of birth is that both your body and your baby seem to know exactly what to do—even if you're a first-time mom. Trusting yourself to listen to the signals your body is sending is half the battle in childbirth. There are also some conscious choices you can make along the way to help make the journey easier for your soon-to-be-born baby.

Gravitational Pull

Obviously if you walk, stand, squat, or assume any other upright position, your baby has the advantages of gravity working for him. Lying prone, whether by choice or by hospital policy, can make your discomfort greater and gives your baby no assistance at all. If you must stay in bed, make sure your head is well elevated so you're in a semisitting or full-sitting position.

Oxygen and Blood Flow

This is where all those breathing exercises you learned in childbirth preparation class come in handy. The air you breathe is giving your baby sufficient oxygen via your bloodstream and is also helping your body and muscles work effectively through contractions. The very process of breathing keeps you centered and focused on the task at hand. Rhythmic breathing can help reduce stress and anxiety, which will make labor pain more manageable and relax your body more readily for birth.

Good Alignment

With that big pregnant belly before you, it's a natural reaction to want to arch your back to counterbalance the weight. But as your mother always told you, stand up straight. Keeping your body in good alignment even before labor begins eases back pain and helps to give your baby the room it needs to move into the proper position for birth. It also allows you to breathe more effectively once labor starts.

Walking Through Labor

While clinical studies have had differing results as to the effectiveness of walking for shortening labor, what is known conclusively is that for many women, walking can ease labor pains and improve their overall satisfaction with their birth experience. It can also give women a greater sense of control and self-empowerment, particularly in a hospital setting. For these reasons, walking is often encouraged. However, staying mobile can be a challenge if your situation requires continuous fetal monitoring, intravenous lines, or any other technology that anchors you to equipment.

Back Labor

Sometimes baby descends with his face toward your abdomen rather than your spine, called the occiput posterior position (OP) or "sunny-side up." The pressure of the head on your coccyx, or tailbone, can cause severe lower back pain, known as back labor.

In addition to the discomfort of back labor, the posterior position can make labor a long and difficult road, because a posterior baby descends straight down with the top of his head, as opposed to an anterior (face down) baby, who tucks in his chin (called flexion) and descends with the smaller back of his head first.

If you are dilated to ten centimeters but are having difficulty pushing out the baby because it is OP, sometimes your health-care provider can turn the baby with her hands or with the help of forceps.

A posterior baby has a much easier job of turning if she hasn't yet engaged significantly into the birth canal. A vaginal exam to check the baby's position in early labor can save much pain and potential interventions (including C-section) by giving you the opportunity to encourage rotation while it's still achievable. Many babies who are OP during labor will spontaneously turn prior to the second stage of labor.

Getting Through Back Labor

Assuming a hands-and-knees position will relieve the pain of back labor (by dropping your uterus away from your spine) and give your baby more room to rotate to an anterior position. Other effective pain-relief methods include massage and counterpressure and warm compresses or water jets (in a shower or whirlpool). Injections of sterile water papules have also been shown to be useful in relieving back labor pain. Your partner could be pre-assigned the job to inquire about these if the case of back labor should present itself.

To try to initiate fetal rotation, your provider may suggest pelvic tilts or rocking, which is simply lifting or rocking your pelvis back and forth while in the hands-and-knees position. The use of pillows or a birthing ball for support can help alleviate strain on your arms and wrists over a long period of time.

Epidurals and Back Labor

While an epidural can provide much-needed pain relief for women experiencing back labor, it also has the potential to worsen the situation by relaxing the uterine floor and potentially allowing the baby to engage further into the pelvis in the posterior position. Talk to your provider now about her strategies for dealing with back labor should it occur.

Time for Rest

Labor can be an exhausting affair, particularly if yours is a long one. If you are completely exhausted by the time you reach the second stage of labor, you may have a difficult time summoning enough strength to push effectively. It's not easy to sleep through contractions, particularly when they start coming close together, but you may be able to grab some small catnaps in between them early on. If you choose to have an epidural or other pharmaceutical pain relief, it can provide a much-needed respite for sleeping and regaining your strength.

Save Your Strength

One way to prevent complete exhaustion during the latter stages of labor is to save your strength early on. It's common for women, especially first-time moms, to want to walk a marathon and mow the lawn at the first twinges of contractions in an effort to speed things along. What often happens instead is that they end up exhausted and unable to marshal their strength when they really need it—during the second stage of labor. While some moderate physical activity is fine, don't overdo it and regret it later.

Once regular contractions begin, take a short nap if your comfort level will allow it. If labor begins in the middle of the night, but contractions are still far apart, try to go back to sleep. At the least, relax and take it easy for a bit, and store up your energy for the big task ahead.

Food and Drink in Labor

The same way rest can help recharge you for birth, taking nourishment can also help fuel your energy stores for the birth process. A light snack and plenty of fluids can keep you hydrated and powered up. If you do eat in labor, light, nonspicy, and easily digestible foods like broth, toast, crackers, and juice are your best bet.

However, given that the majority of laboring women are not in a high-risk situation that would make cesarean and general anesthesia likely, a blanket policy banning food and drink in labor can do more harm than good.

Dehydration, discomfort, mental stress, and ketosis (ketones in the bloodstream) are all potential detrimental effects of banning any oral nourishment in labor. Intravenous fluids are given to help prevent dehydration in women who are not allowed to eat; however, IV fluids are more invasive and have their own set of risks.

Professional opinions on the food and drink issue differ. The American College of Obstetricians and Gynecologists advises that only small sips of water and ice chips be provided to laboring women and that women with long labors be given fluids intravenously, while the American College of Certified Nurse Midwives (ACNM) suggests that midwives allow their low-risk patients to listen to their bodies by "promot[ing] self-determination by healthy women experiencing normal labors as to appropriate intake."

···················· **need to know** ····················

Some hospitals and providers may restrict food and fluid intake because if an emergency situation arises and you require general anesthesia, there is a risk of aspiration of stomach contents, or vomit getting into the lungs.

"NPO" is the clinical acronym for nil per os (Latin for "nothing by mouth"). Hospitals have made NPO the norm for laboring women throughout the latter half of the twentieth century, despite the fact that general anesthesia is rarely used in childbirth today. At the very least, ice chips and water intake should be allowed as comfort measures for low-risk laboring women.

Reflecting these differing philosophies, you'll find that the policies on fluids and food by mouth are generally more liberal in nonhospital settings like the birthing center. Ask your provider and birth facility about their policies on food and drink in labor and the scientific rationale behind them so you can prepare and plan accordingly.

Pushing

Pushing is arguably the hardest task of labor (although some women may say transition is more difficult). Having enough energy to be up to the challenge is the key to effective pushing—another reason why rest in labor is so essential.

If you've had an epidural or other anesthetic block, you will probably need some guidance to push at the right time.

The second stage of labor can last from minutes to hours. Women who have had a previous child usually have a shorter second stage than those who are first-time mothers. Because an epidural or other anesthetic block can make pushing less effective, women who have had an epidural are often allowed more time to push in the second stage of labor.

> **··········· need to know ···········**
>
> The best time for pushing is right at the peak of your contraction. You may be acutely aware of when that is, or you may need a little help from your provider and/or support person to get the timing down.

Vocalization can help you power up your pushing and reserve your strength. Use your voice to strengthen your efforts. Moaning, groaning, or grunting will also "remind" you to breathe, which is important since your baby is still depending on you for oxygen. Take a deep cleansing breath between pushes to keep your energy up. Some women will hold their breath briefly during the push, breathing deeply between contractions. Try not to hold your breath for too long—five seconds is probably a good rule of thumb. You can also try exhaling slowly during your pushes. This type of controlled pushing is less intense and can help prevent perineal tears.

Finally, focus only on the pushing and on seeing your baby. Do not worry about losing control.

··· **need to know** ·························

Women giving birth do urinate, defecate, and pass gas in the process. Your provider is quite used to encountering bodily fluids during the birth process, so don't let self-consciousness inhibit your pushing efforts.

Before you know it, you will be well rewarded for all your hard work.

Birthing Positions

As previously mentioned, getting gravity on your side as you position yourself for birth is an excellent idea. Any upright or semiupright position—standing, leaning, walking, squatting, or sitting—can help move your baby in the right direction.

The rule of thumb in labor positions is if it feels good, do it. Experiment with different stances to see what works best for you. A doula or midwife can also be an invaluable source of suggestions for effective laboring positions. Here are some basic positions to try:

Squatting. Assuming a squatting position, with the support of a person or birthing bar, can increase the diameter of the pelvic outlet and is a natural position for pushing.

Chair sitting. Sitting on a birthing stool, chair, or toilet can help relax your perineum and pelvis.

Kneeling. Getting on your knees and leaning against pillows, your support person, or a chair for support may ease back pain.

Standing or leaning. Staying upright with a partner or support person to lean against can help. Some women find rocking or other rhythmic movement in this position a calming influence.

Squatting is one of the most effective positions you can use in labor and birth. It allows gravity to work in your favor during the pushing phase of labor and opens up your pelvic outlet another one to two centimeters. Just keep in mind that your provider needs to be able to both see and properly support the baby's emerging head to prevent tearing or birth trauma. The use of a birth stool is sometimes helpful in maintaining a squatting position.

If a birthing stool or a squatting bar is not available for you to use as support as you assume a squatting position, a well-placed partner or chair for support can serve the same purpose.

.... **need to know** ....

If you do choose this position for birth, be aware that because it usually shortens the pushing phase and speeds your baby's descent, there is a risk of perineal tearing.

An experienced midwife or birth attendant can often prevent tearing with proper support, however.

The lithotomy, or flat-on-your-back, position is actually quite ineffective for labor and birth. Your heavy uterus is pressing down on the vena cava, a major blood vessel, and potentially lowering your blood pressure and your baby's oxygen supply. You also have no help from gravity. Placing your legs in metal stirrups can make matters worse by putting pressure on your tailbone and narrowing your pelvic outlet. Still, some providers prefer this position because it allows them to see the baby's emerging head better. A modified lithotomy, called McRobert's position, may also be useful in cases of shoulder dystocia by increasing the diameter of your pelvic outlet.

Chapter 14

Labor Management and Intervention

*L*abor and birth pain is in the eye of the beholder, and every woman will have a different perception of just how comfortable her birth experience is. Anxiety and fear over childbirth and anticipated "unbearable" pain can actually make your birth more painful. Fortunately, there are many natural and pharmaceutical options available for soothing labor discomforts.

Choosing Your Weapons

Many first-time moms are under the impression that childbirth is either natural and painful or medicated and tolerable.

Prepared childbirth education classes are an excellent source of information on pain management options and will help you reach an informed decision about which methods you want to try in labor. Talk to other women who have been through birth about what pain-relief methods they found effective. Keep in mind, however, that what was right for them may not necessarily be what you're looking for out of your birth experience.

Breathing Techniques

Breathing can play a very important role in guiding your concentration and making your pain manageable in labor.

Lamaze is a big proponent of patterned breathing. There are several types of breathing taught in Lamaze, each with a different purpose. Breathing techniques are often used in combination with imagery to achieve deeper relaxation. Having a focal point to look at during breathing exercises—either a pleasing photo or simply a chosen place somewhere in the birth room—can help with concentration.

.... **need to know** ....

Most childbirth preparation classes involve some sort of breathing exercises. Practice at home so it becomes second nature by the time your birth arrives.

Lamaze isn't the only childbirth philosophy that teaches controlled respiration; the Bradley Method advocates abdominal breathing for relaxation.

While breathing won't magically eliminate pain, it will give you a greater sense of control, keep you focused and relaxed, and make the pain more manageable.

Systemic Analgesics

Analgesics work by depressing the nervous system and therefore lessening the sensation of pain. They do not render you unconscious, although they may render you silly. The narcotics meperidine (Demerol), nalbuphine (Nubain), butorphanol (Stadol), and fentanyl (Sublimaze) are all analgesic drugs that are commonly used to relieve labor pain.

····· **need to know** ·····

An analgesic reduces pain but doesn't eliminate it completely, while an anesthetic removes sensation, and therefore pain, completely. Both can be effective tools in management of labor pain.

Analgesics are administered as an injection. When used at the right point in labor and in the correct dosage, analgesics will not cause your baby any serious side effects. However, because analgesics do cross the placenta, the administration of narcotics too late in labor can cause sluggishness in baby that can result in low blood oxygen levels and difficulty latching on and sucking during afterbirth breastfeeding attempts. They can also decrease normal variability patterns in the fetal heart rate.

Blocks and Epidurals

Regional anesthesia is a drug that numbs or deadens the sensation in a specific portion of the body. Unlike narcotics, which can make you feel sleepy or stoned, a regional anesthetic like a spinal block or epidural leaves you mentally alert. According to the Mayo Clinic, an estimated 2.4 million women who give birth in the Unites States each year receive an epidural for pain management.

Because epidurals and blocks can slow labor, some providers may strongly suggest that you reach a certain dilation benchmark (usually four to five centimeters) before receiving one. However, ACOG has issued a statement saying that the standard of practice should be that an epidural is never denied to any woman in labor who requests one for pain control, no matter how far she is dilated. Women who have their labor induced may have more severe contractions before significant dilation even occurs and often find a need for epidural relief well before the four-centimeter mark. It's a good idea to discuss any concerns about epidural timing with your health-care provider before the birth.

Lumbar Epidural

The most common type of regional anesthetic used in labor is a lumbar epidural, which temporarily deadens the nerves from your navel to your knees. If you decide to have an epidural, an anesthesiologist will be called in to administer it. The procedure takes just a few minutes to complete. You will be asked to roll over on your side or sit at the edge of the bed to expose your lower back, which will be swabbed with an antiseptic solution to prevent infection. The anesthesiologist will then insert a thin plastic catheter into the area between your fourth and fifth vertebrae, which is called the epidural space. Once in place, the catheter is taped down and the anesthetic is injected into it. You can then assume a more comfortable position.

There are a variety of regional anesthetics that can be used in epidurals for labor and birth; two of the most common drugs are bupivacaine (Sensorcaine) and ropivacaine (Naropin). The anesthetics work by blocking the nerve impulses that regulate sensation and pain. They are sometimes administered in combination with epinephrine, which speeds the onset and prolongs the efficacy of the anesthetic, or with a narcotic analgesic such as fentanyl (Sublimaze).

If you weren't hooked up to an intravenous line and saline drip already, one will be started prior to the epidural. The epidural can cause hypotension (low blood pressure), so having the IV in place cannot only keep your fluid volume up but also provides easy access for an injection of drugs to treat you should your blood pressure drop dangerously low. You will also be encouraged to keep your head elevated, as lying flat on your back could make hypotension worse. If you were not having continuous fetal monitoring before the epidural, you will start now.

A lumbar epidural takes about twenty minutes to fully take effect. Once it does, the numbness lasts several hours. While the epidural deadens the nerves, it has no effect on the involuntary muscles that control your contractions, which will continue even though you may now be blissfully unaware of them.

Walking Epidurals

For those who want the pain relief of an epidural, but aren't interested in being confined to their hospital beds, there is an option. A low-dose combined spinal epidural, more commonly known as a walking epidural, numbs the same area as a standard lumbar epidural but allows you to retain enough sensation to move around and walk. This type of epidural is administered with a fine needle that is guided through the epidural catheter and into the spinal fluid (not the epidural space), where anesthetic medication is injected.

Spinal Block

A spinal block is used in cesarean delivery to numb the area from your waist down. A dose of anesthetic is injected into your lower back into the fluid-filled space that cushions your spinal column, known as the intrathecal space (a spinal block is sometimes called an intrathecal for this reason). Much faster than an epidural, a spinal block takes effect almost immediately. Spinal block may also be used in cases of an assisted birth to relieve any pain associated with forceps use.

Possible Pitfalls

So are there downsides to an epidural? Some clinical studies have found that the first and second stages of labor are often prolonged with an epidural, especially in women who are giving birth for the first time. However, other studies have not noted a statistically significant difference in labor times for women having an epidural, so further research is needed to investigate any adverse effects of epidurals on length of labor.

As with any procedure that punctures the skin, there is a risk of infection with an epidural or a spinal block.

There is conflicting evidence as to whether or not epidural use increases your chance of cesarean; some retrospective studies have found an association, while other studies have not.

Another potential drawback is the possibility of a postdural puncture headache (often called a PDPH). This severe headache occurs when the dura that sheaths the cerebral spinal fluid (CSF) around the spinal column is unintentionally punctured and fluid starts to leak into the epidural space. The resulting drop in spinal fluid pressure is what triggers the headache, which usually gets worse upon standing.

Postdural puncture headache is more common in spinal blocks because it is easier for the dura to be unintentionally punctured in that procedure.

However, the size and type of needle used and the technique with which the needle insertion is done have an influence on whether or not you develop CSF leakage. If you do get a PDPH, rest and rehydration can usually resolve the problem. In some cases an injection of blood into the epidural space, called a blood patch, may be required to seal the puncture site and stop the leakage.

Other Regional Blocks

Other less common regional blocks sometimes used to relieve labor pain include a paracervical block, which involves an injection into your cervix, and a caudal block, which is injected into the tailbone and numbs your abdominal and pelvic muscles.

In situations when your baby needs a little help coming out, you may be a candidate for another type of regional anesthetic block used at delivery. A pudendal block, which deadens the nerves in the pelvic floor and vagina, or a saddle block, which numbs your perineum, bottom, and inner thighs, may be given to provide pain relief if an episiotomy or a forceps or vacuum extraction is required.

Give Yourself Choices

As you can see, every method of pain relief has its pros and cons. You must weigh the risks and benefits in light of your particular birth needs. You may have made some general decisions about how you'd like to handle labor pain on the birth day but give yourself permission to change your mind—without guilt—at any time. For first-time moms, making a cast-in-stone commitment to one pain-management method now is like buying a car without a test drive. And even if you've been through labor and delivery before, this time around may be completely different.

Along with pain relief options, a twenty-first century woman has a dizzying array of technology at her disposal to employ in the birth process. Yet labor and birth remain, in essence, completely natural processes that women have been experiencing forever without the aid of monitors, synthetic induction, or extraction tools. Knowing what is available, and more importantly, when interventions are necessary versus when they are simply prophylactic, is essential to making informed decisions at your birth.

Informed Consent

In simplest terms, informed consent is making sure you as a patient fully understand a given medical intervention and any risks associated with it well enough to make an informed decision on whether or not to agree to the procedure. Unless you are mentally or physically incapacitated for some unforeseen reason, you ultimately have the final say on what interventions are used or not used in your birth.

Ideally, informed consent is a process made up of three major steps.

1. **Education.** Your provider should objectively brief you on exactly what the intervention entails, and explain the risks and benefits to the procedure in laymen's terms.

2. **Alternatives.** Your provider should inform you of any possible alternatives to the intervention, along with the pros and cons of each.

3. **Assessment.** Your provider should ensure that you've understood everything that was just explained and ask if you have any questions before you make your decision.

In practice, the process of obtaining informed consent may be colored by a provider's own beliefs or personal agenda, either consciously or subconsciously. Fears of malpractice or liability issues, provider care preferences, and even scheduling issues can influence the process. This is why it is so important for a woman to learn all she can about the pros and cons of interventional procedures before birth. Informed consent is much easier to give, or deny, if your first lesson about a given procedure happens well before birth rather than in a potentially stressful environment or emergency situation.

················· **need to know** ·······················

When you are preparing your birth plan, keep in mind that unexpected emergencies may come up.

Along with educating yourself about emergency procedures, don't be afraid to ask your provider about potential situations and come up with possible game plans. A frank discussion about birth plans should always include mention of the fact that no one can predict what will happen, and that last-minute changes of plan are not uncommon.

Preparatory Procedures

Intervention choices may begin in early in labor when you first enter a birth facility. Prepping procedures will vary depending on facility policy and your provider's preferences. The following sections discuss some prep procedures that you may potentially encounter.

To Shave or Not to Shave

Although the practice is much less common than it once was, a few hospitals still perform a shave of the perineal and/or pubic area. The rationale is that it improves visibility and minimizes infection. If your hospital advocates the shaving routine and you'd rather avoid being shaved, you can either do it at home yourself, if you prefer, or discuss the possibility of not having this largely unnecessary procedure.

Formal Attire

If giving birth at a hospital, you'll be handed that old favorite, the backdraft hospital gown, to put on after admission. While the back opening can allow an anesthesiologist easy access for an epidural or other anesthetic block, it can be uncomfortable and embarrassing for many women. Ask about wearing your own nightgown from home, or bring a robe along for extra coverage.

Enema Anyone?

An enema before birth can help clean out your bowels and theoretically will make the trip down the birth canal easier for your little one, which is why some hospitals still use them as part of their prepping procedure. However, enemas can also be uncomfortable and unnecessary. The fact is that contractions will naturally loosen your bowels, and many women have spent a great deal of time on the toilet already during early labor, emptying them the standard way. If you feel you don't really need an enema and the hospital offers one, explain that you're already covered in that department.

Locks and Lines

Some hospitals may insert what is known as a heparin or saline lock into your arm as standard procedure. The lock is simply a needle encased in a plastic hub that is inserted into a vein and attached to your arm with surgical tape. A small amount of saline or heparin, a blood thinner, is then flushed through the lock to prevent clotting. If intravenous medication is suddenly needed in labor, the lock provides easy access. An intravenous line, or IV, can be attached to the lock at any point. If you have the lock on for more than eight hours without any attached tubing, it may be flushed periodically to prevent clotting.

Other facilities may start you on an IV at admission to keep you hydrated. Medication can also be added to the IV if necessary. If yours isn't considered a high-risk birth and you don't want an IV, there's really no reason you can't hydrate yourself the old-fashioned way—by drinking fluids.

In addition, if a glucose drip is given to a laboring mother, there is an increased risk of hypoglycemia (low blood sugar) for the baby at birth. It can also cause electrolyte imbalances such as hyponatremia (sodium depletion), in mother and child. Any type of intravenous fluid drip also introduces a risk of fluid overload in a laboring woman if not managed properly.

Finally, if you're having a cesarean section or having an epidural or another type of anesthetic block that will give you no muscle control over your urine flow, you'll require a urinary catheter.

A full bladder in labor can keep your baby from descending properly, as well as being just plain uncomfortable. If you can and wish to make it to the bathroom on your own, include that in your birth plan.

Fetal Monitoring

During labor, an electronic fetal monitor is used to monitor your baby's heart rate (fetal heart rate, or FHR) and your contractions (uterine activity, or UA) to ensure that labor is progressing normally. The monitor will also alert your provider to excessive fetal stress from oxygen deprivation or umbilical cord problems. Some fetal monitoring units measure your blood pressure and heart rate as well as fetal blood oxygen levels.

On the down side, continuous electronic fetal monitoring has been associated with an increased incidence of C-section and operative delivery such as forceps or episiotomy birth, and all the associated risks of those procedures.

If you're having a home or birthing center birth, you may have the option of having your baby's heart rate monitored with a fetoscope, a stethoscope, or a handheld Doppler device like the one your provider may have used during prenatal checkups. Using these devices, the FHR is taken after a contraction, and your provider will monitor it for a full minute, counting the beats in each five-second interval until he has twelve sets of five-second FHR samples to ensure that the variability of the heart rate is "reassuring." This technique, called intermittent auscultation, may be preferred by women who don't like the restrictions of traditional electronic fetal monitoring.

Internal and External

With external fetal monitoring, two belts are positioned on your abdomen—one low and one higher—to measure the FHR and UA. A small sensor called a transducer is on the skin-side of each of the belts. The transducers pick up the heartbeat and contractions and transfer the information back to the base unit.

The base unit provides a visual representation of the FHR and your contractions on a computer screen. The base unit may also print out a paper strip of tracings that provides a hard copy of the progress of your labor, a good practice if health-care providers are attending to other labors and are in and out of your birth room.

If you are given oxytocin (Pitocin) to induce labor or strengthen contractions, it's quite possible the provider and/or facility will require continuous fetal monitoring, which will keep you in bed. Again, talk to your provider well in advance of your due date so if oxytocin is offered during your birth, you'll know the potential perks and pitfalls.

If yours is a high-risk pregnancy and your amniotic sac has broken, an internal monitor may be recommended. An internal monitor uses the same base unit, but instead of belt transducers, a tiny springlike coil of wire is inserted vaginally. The coil is inserted just under the skin on the baby's scalp and provides an electrocardiographic (ECG) analysis of the FHR. Internal monitoring is almost exclusively used in a hospital setting, and women who are internally monitored are generally restricted to their beds. If you have concerns about the possibility of internal monitoring, talk with your provider about the circumstances under which it might be required and what your options are.

Episiotomy

Episiotomy is the surgical incision of the perineum—the area between your vagina and your anus—to facilitate the passage of your baby's head during the final pushing stage of birth. The perineum, however, is an amazingly pliable piece of tissue, and the majority of women find it can stretch to accommodate their babies' heads without the need of episiotomy.

Several studies have shown a dramatic drop in episiotomy rates since the early 1980s, yet episiotomy continues to be one of the most frequently performed surgical procedures that women undergo. The ACOG does not endorse the practice of "routine episiotomy" without valid medical indications.

Types of Episiotomy

The midline episiotomy involves an incision from the vagina out toward the anus. The mediolateral episiotomy uses an incision that starts at the vagina but extends out diagonally instead of directly toward the anus to avoid rectal tearing. The size of both episiotomy incisions and perineal tears are referred to in degrees to indicate their severity. A first-degree tear would be the most superficial, and a fourth-degree the most severe.

Preventing Perineal Tears

The use of warm (not hot) compresses on the perineum and perineal massage in the final weeks of pregnancy can help the stretching process along and avoid perineal tears. Controlled pushing during the second stage of labor can also keep your perineum intact, as can provider support of the head and perineal tissues if the baby is crowning too quickly. If you don't want an episiotomy, talk to your provider about your wishes and include that point in your birth plan.

Before birth, you can help prepare your perineum for the big day by massaging the perineal area with oils or lubricant and by practicing kegel exercises. Kegels exercise the pelvic floor muscles and can help you with more controlled pushing during the birth. They also help to avoid urinary incontinence. To do kegels, repeatedly tighten and relax the muscles you use to start and stop urine flow.

.... **need to know** ....

There may be some situations in which an episiotomy is unavoidable, such as when a forceps or vacuum extraction delivery is medically required or your baby is in distress and needs to be delivered quickly.

One of the common misconceptions about episiotomy is that it prevents urinary and/or fecal incontinence later in life. However, the truth is that the routine use of episiotomy can actually increase the chance of that complication. A 2003 metanalysis of the episiotomy literature in the journal *Urology* found that routine midline episiotomy increases the risk of serious perineal lacerations, which may lead to fecal incontinence, and routine mediolateral episiotomy does nothing to prevent urinary incontinence (UI) or severe perineal tears.

A 2002 study in the journal *Birth* that reviewed national birth data from the National Center for Health Statistics found that episiotomies are more likely to develop into more severe lacerations (that is, third and fourth degree) than natural tears of the perineum in women who don't have the procedure, which are usually first or second degree.

If an episiotomy is done, or if tearing does occur, you will receive stitches after the birth to close up the lacerations. An anesthetic block will be injected first if you haven't already had one. You may also receive postpartum antibiotic therapy depending on the degree of the tear or incision.

Chapter 15

Breastfeeding Basics

*G*ood nutrition for your little one right from the start will get him off to a healthy beginning. Breastmilk or formula is the only food your infant needs for his first four to six months of life. If you decide to breastfeed, following some sound nutritional guidelines can ensure you are getting all of the calories and nutrients needed to nourish your baby properly.

Why Breastfeed?

One of the very first decisions new parents make is how to feed their newborn. Many health professionals agree that the ideal method is breastfeeding, though for some women this is not the best choice for physical, health, or personal reasons. For some mothers, breastfeeding is an easy transition. For others it may take some time and patience before the process is a smooth one. It is perfectly normal for it to take some time and practice. A lactation consultant should visit you in the hospital to help you get started.

The American Dietetic Association (ADA) and the American Academy of Pediatrics (AAP) both recommend that babies be breastfed exclusively for the first four to six months of life and then breastfed with complementary foods for at least twelve months.

Benefits of Breastfeeding

Even though breastfeeding is not your only option, there are many benefits to using this method to nourish your newborn in the beginning. Breastfeeding can aid in the physical, emotional, and practical needs of both the baby and the mother. Other benefits include these:

- The infant is able to eat on demand without any trouble. When the infant is hungry, the milk is ready instantly without any measuring, mixing, or warming of bottles.
- There is no concern over proper sterilization.
- Breastmilk is easy for babies to digest, so there is less spitting up.
- Breastmilk is rich in antibodies that can help protect the baby from intestinal, ear, urinary, and lower respiratory-tract infections, as well as pneumonia.
- If breastfeeding is continued through at least the first six months of life, it can help decrease the risk of the baby's developing food allergies.
- In babies with a family history of food allergies, breastfeeding can help lower the risk of developing asthma and some skin conditions.

- The quality and the quantity of fat in breastmilk tends to be more nutritious than the fat found in most formulas.
- Breastfeeding is less expensive than formula feeding.
- New studies indicate that breastfed infants may be less likely to become obese later in life and therefore less likely to develop diabetes.
- Women who breastfeed usually return to their prepregnancy weight more quickly, and the uterus also returns to its normal size more quickly.
- Breastfeeding can help reduce the risk of ovarian cancer and, in premenopausal women, breast cancer.

How the Body Produces Breastmilk

In the first few days after birth, a woman's body produces a fluid called colostrum. This is the first milk that the infant receives. Colostrum is a thick, yellowish substance that is produced just prior to the flow of breastmilk. It contains antibodies and immunoglobulins, which help protect the newborn from bacteria and viruses and help to prevent the infant's immature gut from becoming infected. Colostrum is high in protein, zinc, and other minerals and contains less fat, carbohydrates, and calories than actual breastmilk.

Between the third and sixth day after birth, colostrum begins to change to a "transitional" form of breastmilk. During this time, the amounts of protein and immune factors in the milk gradually decrease while fat, lactose, and calories in the milk increase. By about the tenth day after birth, the mother begins to produce mature breastmilk. One of the special qualities of breastmilk is its ability to change to meet the needs of your growing baby throughout the course of breastfeeding.

················· **need to know** ·························

The size of breasts is not a factor in how much milk a mother produces. Instead it is the infant's feeding habits that control milk production.

In other words, the more a woman breastfeeds her infant, the more milk her body will produce.

The Nutrition of Breastmilk

At this point, human breastmilk provides the most optimal nutrition for infants. Breastmilk seems to have the perfect balance of carbohydrates, fats, and proteins as well as vitamins and minerals that the infant needs. Breastmilk contains just enough protein to keep from overloading the baby's immature kidneys. The fat in breastmilk is also easily absorbed by an infant's digestive system. Breastmilk provides liberal amounts of vital essential fatty acids, saturated fats, triglycerides, and cholesterol. It contains long-chain polyunsaturated fatty acids that are essential for proper development of the central nervous system. Breastmilk is relatively low in sodium and provides adequate amounts of minerals such as zinc, iron, and calcium, which reduce the demand for these nutrients from the mother.

Breastmilk contains large amounts of lactose, or milk sugar. Lactose is utilized in the tissues of the brain and spinal cord and helps to provide the infant with energy. Breastmilk contains only a small amount of iron, but the iron is in a form that is readily absorbed. Fifty percent of the iron in breastmilk is absorbed, compared with only 4 to 10 percent of the iron in cow's milk or commercial infant formula.

The ABCs of Breastfeeding

Proper technique is important to make sure the process goes smoothly and the baby consumes enough milk. In addition to techniques, you will have plenty of questions as to how much, when, and how long. Take the time to get the advice, support, education, and encouragement you need from a lactation consultant, pediatrician, family, friends, and support groups.

········· **need to know** ·········

Breastfeeding requires much commitment from the mother. If you choose to go back to work outside of the home or if you are separated from your infant for other reasons, a breast pump can be used to collect breastmilk when needed.

How Often to Breastfeed

Babies who are breastfed tend to feed more often than babies who are formula fed. Breastfed babies generally eat eight to twelve times per day.

This is basically because breastfed babies' stomachs empty more quickly since breastmilk is so easy to digest. The baby should eat until she is full, usually ten to fifteen minutes per breast. At first, most newborns want to eat every few hours, both during the day and at night. Babies generally eat on demand when they are hungry.

Look for signs from your baby that she is hungry, such as increased alertness or activity, mouthing, or rooting around the breast. Crying seems to be more of a later sign of hunger. As your baby gets older and becomes alert for longer periods of time, you can more easily settle into a routine schedule of feeding every three hours or so with fewer sessions at night. By the end of the first month, babies will generally start sleeping longer throughout the night.

Is My Baby Getting Enough Milk?

A worry for many breastfeeding moms is whether the newborn is getting enough to eat. With formulas, you are able to tell exactly how many ounces the baby has consumed, but with breastfeeding this is harder to identify. It may seem at first that the baby is hungry all the time, which makes some moms wonder if he has had enough. This is completely normal. Babies should be hungry quite often because breastmilk is digested within a couple of hours after consumption. After the baby's first few days of life, he will want to nurse about eight to twelve times per day. The baby should be fed on demand, with no worry about schedules, until you have breastfeeding down pat and can begin to recognize your baby's own schedule. The baby's pediatrician will be able to tell if your baby is getting enough to eat by how much weight he gains at each visit.

There are other ways to tell if your baby is getting enough to eat. After the fifth day of birth, she should have at least six to eight wet diapers per day and three to four loose yellow stools per day. She is most likely getting enough if she is nursing at least ten to fifteen minutes on each breast. Your baby should show steady weight gain after the first week of age. Her urine should be pale yellow and not deep yellow or orange. You should find your baby wanting to eat at least every two to three hours or at least eight times per day for at least the first two to three weeks. In addition, she should have good skin color. If you become concerned about whether your baby is getting enough to eat, contact your pediatrician or lactation consultant. Babies who are not getting enough to eat can become easily dehydrated.

In general, most babies lose a little weight, 5 to 10 percent of their birth weight, in their first few days of life. They should start to gain at least one ounce per day by the fifth day after birth and be back to their birth weight by two weeks after birth.

Is Breastmilk Enough?

During the first six months of life, most babies who are breastfeeding will not require any additional water, juices, vitamins, iron, or formula. With sound breastfeeding practices, supplements are rarely needed because breastmilk provides the infant with just about all the fluids and nutrients he needs for proper growth and development. By six months of age, it is generally recommended that babies be introduced to foods that contain iron in addition to breastmilk.

While the water supply in most U.S. cities and towns contains plenty of fluoride, a mineral often found in tap water that is important for strong teeth and prevention of cavities, in certain rural areas the levels can be too low. Breastmilk contains very low levels of fluoride. However, babies under six months of age should not be given fluoride supplements, even if levels in your water supply are low.

Vitamin D Controversy

Though breastmilk is a complete source of nutrition for your baby, there is some controversy surrounding the need for supplementing with vitamin D. Vitamin D is found in only small amounts in breastmilk and is necessary to absorb calcium into the bones and teeth. However, the vitamin D in breastmilk is in a very absorbable form and therefore is generally adequate for most infants. Babies who may be at higher risk for vitamin D deficiency include those who have little exposure to sunlight. Moderate sunlight helps to produce vitamin D in the body, and mother and babies with darker skin may have a harder time getting enough sunlight to produce vitamin D.

Mothers deficient in vitamin D also create a risk of low levels in their babies. The amount of vitamin D in breastmilk is directly related to the level of vitamin D in the mother's body. If you are taking a prenatal or vitamin/mineral supplement that contains vitamin D, drinking milk, and getting moderate exposure to sunlight, your breastmilk should contain optimal levels of vitamin D. The American Academy of Pediatrics recently began recommending that all infants, including those who are exclusively breastfed, have a minimum intake of 200 international units (IU) of vitamin D per day beginning in the first two months of life.

Other Concerns

Babies sometimes react to certain foods that the mother eats because they may pass through to the breastmilk. After eating spicy or gassy foods, the mother may notice the baby crying or fussing as well as nursing more often. However, these symptoms may also show up in babies with colic. You will know it is a reaction to food you have eaten if the symptoms last less than twenty-four hours. Symptoms caused by colic generally occur daily and often last for days or weeks at a time. If your baby seems to react to certain foods that you eat, eliminate those foods from your diet. There is no need to eliminate foods from your diet unless you have a specific reason to suspect a particular food is bothering your baby. If you have a family history of allergies, including asthma, you may want to avoid foods you are allergic or sensitive to while breastfeeding.

···················· **need to know** ····················

The American Academy of Pediatrics suggests that breastfeeding mothers of susceptible infants (with a family history of allergies) are wise to eliminate peanuts and peanut-containing foods while breastfeeding.

Although the reaction is rare, some babies are allergic to cow's milk and foods that contain cow's milk in the mother's diet. Symptoms will usually appear a few minutes to a few hours after a breastfeeding session. They can include diarrhea, rash, fussiness, gas, runny nose, cough, or congestion. Talk to your pediatrician if your baby experiences any of these symptoms. Other foods you consume that may cause reactions in your newborn include chocolate, citrus fruits and juices, and common food allergens such as eggs, wheat, corn, fish, nuts, and soy.

Nutritional Requirements for the Breastfeeding Mom

As with pregnancy, it is vital that a mother eat a healthy, well-balanced diet to ensure that she gets all of the nutrients she needs for successful breastfeeding. The mother's diet needs to fulfill her own nutritional needs as well as additional needs, which increase during breastfeeding. At this time your body's first priority is milk production, and if you lack the right type of nourishment in your diet, your personal needs may not be met.

Calorie Needs

Your body's fuel supply for milk production comes from two main sources: extra calories, or energy, from foods you eat and energy stored as body fat during pregnancy.

·················· **need to know** ··················

For your body to produce breastmilk, it uses about 100 to 150 calories a day from fat that your body naturally stored during pregnancy. That is why breastfeeding moms often lose pregnancy weight more quickly.

In addition, you also need to eat about 500 extra calories per day (or 500 calories more than your maintenance calorie level) during breastfeeding. In general, consuming 500 extra calories per day than before pregnancy will meet your energy needs for breastmilk production.

Figuring on light to moderate activity, on average a woman needs about 2,700 calories per day. You need more calories if you are a teenager or more active. You can easily get these extra calories by eating nutritious foods from all of the food groups in the Food Guide Pyramid. The following number of servings from the Food Guide Pyramid would provide about 2,700 calories.

- 10 servings from the bread, cereal, rice, and pasta group (choose whole grains and whole-wheat products more often)
- 4 servings from the vegetable group
- 4 servings from the fruit group
- 3–4 servings of dairy (choose nonfat or low-fat dairy products). Teens should shoot for 4 servings per day
- 2 servings (6–7 ounces) from the meat, poultry, fish, dry beans, eggs, and nut group (choose leaner meats more often as well as occasionally choose nonmeat selections such as legumes, nuts, or seeds)
- Use fats and sweets sparingly

Once breastfeeding is well established, a mother can reduce the number of excess calories modestly. This will increase the rate the body uses stored fat without an adverse impact on breastmilk production. Be cautious not to cut calories drastically during breastfeeding, which can reduce daily milk production.

How to Fuel Your Body

While you are breastfeeding, it is still important to remember that you are still eating for two. You need to continue the healthy diet you followed during pregnancy through breastfeeding and beyond. Not only is it important to get extra calories, but those extra calories need to come from healthy foods. Eating a healthy, well-balanced diet will ensure you are getting the carbohydrates, protein, and healthy fats you need for breastfeeding.

Focus on fueling your body with whole-grain starches, fresh fruits and vegetables, and lean protein foods that will provide plenty of protein, calcium, and iron.

Eating a variety of foods is important because this way, you can be sure to obtain different nutrients. Eating in moderation is the key, not too much of any one food or item.

Rapid weight loss and cutting calories too low can pose a danger to your baby. Since milk production requires extra calorie expenditure, even increasing your caloric level by 500 calories will allow for a safe amount of weight loss. Losing weight gradually through a healthy, well-balanced diet and regular exercise is the safest route.

Nutrient Needs of the Breastfeeding Mom

The process of breastfeeding is nutritionally demanding for a mother. During breastfeeding your need for many nutrients will increase even more than during pregnancy. The amount of milk you produce is not likely affected by the food you consume, unless you cut your calories drastically.

However, the composition of your milk may vary with certain nutrients depending on your dietary intake.

Calcium

Though your calcium needs don't change during breastfeeding, calcium is still an important nutrient during this time. The recommended amount of 1,000 mg for women over nineteen is a must. If you come up short, your body may draw from the calcium reserves in your bones, which can put you at greater risk for osteoporosis later in life. It can also cause periodontal problems down the line. In addition to dairy foods, choose other foods high in calcium such as dark-green leafy vegetables, fish with edible bones, almonds, and fortified beverages.

B Vitamins

A few of the B vitamins deserve special mention, including vitamin B12, folic acid, and vitamin B6. The daily recommended intake for vitamin B12 increases slightly during breastfeeding. If you are a strict vegetarian, your breastmilk might be missing adequate stores of vitamin B12. Ensure your prenatal or multivitamin contains adequate amounts of vitamin B12. If you are not a vegetarian, you most likely are getting enough. Folic acid, another B vitamin, is important especially if you are considering another pregnancy soon. Vitamin B6 increases slightly during breastfeeding, and women often do not consume enough. Chicken, fish, and pork are great sources of this B vitamin as well as whole-grain products and legumes.

Iron

Iron requirements are lower after your baby is born and you are breast-feeding. The needs go down to 9 mg per day for adult women until you begin to menstruate again, in which case needs go back to normal (18 mg per day). If you are taking an iron supplement, it will not increase iron levels in your breastmilk. Anemia in nursing moms has been associated with decreased milk supply. If you are anemic, you should speak to your doctor about a safe dosage of iron supplementation. You can often improve your condition by making changes to your diet. Including foods with absorb-able iron sources and including a source of vitamin C with these foods can help to bring up your iron levels.

Zinc

Zinc requirements only increase slightly from pregnancy to breastfeed-ing. You lose some zinc when breastfeeding, and your diet may not always be able to compensate for the loss. If you are taking a prenatal or multivita-min, it should take care of any zinc requirements you may not be getting.

Supplements During Breastfeeding

Some doctors may recommend continuing your prenatal supplement through breastfeeding. You can get enough nutrients through the foods you eat if you consistently make good choices. If you come up short on your calories or nutrients, your breastmilk is usually still sufficient for support-ing your baby's proper growth and development. Unless you are severely malnourished, your breastmilk will provide what the infant requires. However, this will be at the expense of your own nutrient reserves. Keep in mind that vitamin and mineral supplements should never be used to make up for poor eating habits.

Essential Fluids

You need to drink lots of fluids and stay well hydrated while breastfeeding. A hormone called oxytocin that is released by your body during breastfeeding tends to make you thirsty. Although fluids will not directly affect your milk supply, it is still recommended to drink at least eight to twelve glasses of water each day.

Harmful Substances

As with pregnancy, it is essential to think about all the substances you put into your body that can pass through to your breastmilk and on to your baby. Many medications are safe to take during breastfeeding, but a few, including herbal products and/or supplements, can be dangerous to your infant.

••••••••••••••••••••••••• **need to know** •••••••••••••••••••••••••

Always get approval from your doctor before taking any prescription or over-the-counter medications while breastfeeding.

Alcohol should be avoided because it can pass through your breastmilk to the baby. You would be wise to cut back on caffeine due to the fact that it can build up in a baby's system. A cup or two a day of coffee or cola is not likely to do harm, but too much can lead to problems. The guidelines for eating fish (due to mercury levels, as discussed in Chapter 7) also pertain to women who are breastfeeding. Habits such as smoking and illegal drugs can cause a mother to produce less milk, and chemicals such as nicotine can pass through the breastmilk.

Formula Feeding

Don't beat yourself up if you cannot breastfeed for some reason. Many women cannot breastfeed for medical, physical, or other reasons. If you are not able to breastfeed or choose not to, today's infant formulas do provide a good nutritious alternative. Most are manufactured in a way that closely mimics, as much as possible, the components of breastmilk. They are made to be easy for babies to digest and provide all of the nutrition needed. It is virtually impossible for a mother to create a formula at home that would have the same complex combination of proteins, sugars, fats, vitamins, and minerals that a baby needs and that are present in commercial formulas and breastmilk. Therefore, if you do not breastfeed your baby, you should use only a commercially prepared formula.

Because of its contents, cow's milk is not appropriate for infants younger than twelve months. Although some formulas are cow-milk based, they have been modified to meet an infant's special needs.

What's in Formula?

Commercial formulas are usually cow-milk based and are fortified with iron as well as other essential vitamins and minerals. Some manufacturers even include some substances found directly in breastmilk that can be manufactured. For infants who cannot tolerate cow's milk, there are also soy-based formulas. Formula feeding is more costly than breastfeeding but, on the other hand, is more convenient for some mothers. Today's commercial formula products are manufactured under strict sterile conditions, so there is no worry about contamination.

Iron-fortified infant formulas have been credited for the declining incidence of iron deficiency anemia in infants. For this reason, the American Academy of Pediatrics highly recommends that mothers who are not breastfeeding use an iron-fortified infant formula.

The Pros and Cons

Some women feel that formula-feeding their infant gives them a little more freedom and that other members of the family, such as the father, can be more active in the feeding and caring of the infant.

Just as breastfeeding has its own unique demands, so does formula feeding. The main demands of formula feeding are organization, handling, and proper preparation. You need to make sure to have enough formula on hand, and bottles must be prepared very carefully using sterile methods. The bottles and nipples must be kept sanitary and ready for when you need them.

Preparing Formulas

Commercial formulas come in all types of varieties. There are ready-to-feed liquids, concentrated liquids that require diluting with water, and powders that require mixing with water. You should always follow closely the instructions on the label for preparing bottles. As well as varieties of formulas, there are many different types of bottles and nipples available to choose from. You may need to experiment with a few different brands before you find a combination that works best for you and your baby.

Bottles should be warmed just slightly before feeding.

··········· **need to know** ··········

Never heat a bottle of formula in a microwave! The formula can heat unevenly and leave hot spots, which can burn a baby's mouth. A microwave can also heat the formula too much, making it too hot for an infant's mouth.

The best way is to heat water in the microwave, take the water out, and then heat the bottle in the water. Always test the formula to make sure the temperature is not too hot. Always wash bottles and nipples thoroughly in hot water, and wash your hands before preparing them.

Do not leave bottles out of the refrigerator for longer than one hour. If your baby doesn't finish a bottle, the contents should be discarded. If formula bottles are prepared in advance, they should be stored in the refrigerator for no longer than twenty-four hours.

breastfeeding basics

How Often to Formula Feed

Experts agree that for the first few weeks, you shouldn't try to follow too rigid a feeding schedule. As the baby gets older, you may be able to work out a more established schedule. You should offer a bottle every two to three hours at first as you see signs of hunger. Until she reaches about ten pounds, she will probably take approximately two to three ounces per feeding. From there, intake will gradually increase. Don't force her to eat if she does not seem hungry. You may see certain signs when the baby has enough such as, closing her mouth or turning away from the bottle, falling asleep, fussiness, and biting or playing with the bottle's nipple. One advantage to bottle feeding is that you can know exactly how much your baby is eating. Your pediatrician can advise you on optimal amounts to feed your baby as she grows.

Chapter 16

Your Baby's Here!

The first days at home with your new family are fun but challenging. Your body is going through some intense physical changes. And if you thought those hormonal changes that pregnancy brought were now finished, well, think again. Enjoy this special time getting acquainted and settling into your new lifestyle.

Your Body Postpartum

From the moment your child slides out of your body, a transformation as dramatic as that of pregnancy begins. Right at delivery you will drop around ten to fifteen pounds of baby, placenta, amniotic fluid, and lochia.

········· **need to know** ·························

By the tenth day postpartum, your incredible shrinking uterus will have contracted to one-twentieth of its prelabor size and the cervix will be closed once again.

Afterpains similar to menstrual cramps and a steady discharge of lochia indicate that the uterus is returning to normal. The lochia flow will continue up to six weeks, but the afterpains will probably stop several days after delivery (although nursing may continue to stimulate them periodically). Your perineal area may continue to be sore for a few weeks, particularly when you need to relieve yourself. Take your peribottle from the hospital home with you and keep it in the bathroom for regular use. A hot water bottle and occasional cold packs can also ease pain and swelling. If sitting is uncomfortable, you can purchase a foam "donut" for your chair at a medical supply store.

As your body drops tissue, fluids, and decreases its cardiovascular volume, your metabolism may seem completely out of whack. Vaginally, things may seem a little "looser" in general. Your vaginal skin is quite elastic and may be stretched out from the birth. Exercise and time will help it return to a firmer state. Constipation is another common postpartum problem, primarily because of the loss of abdominal muscle tone and painkillers that can slow your digestive processes. Plenty of water, movement, and high-fiber foods may help. If you had a C-section, your incision may also make you hesitant to bear down very hard. Supporting it with a rolled up towel can help. A stool softener may be prescribed as well; check with your practitioner if you are breastfeeding before taking any medication.

Your breasts will be tender as you deal with engorgement. Women who aren't planning on nursing will find that drying up your milk supply fully can be a somewhat uncomfortable process. If you do breastfeed, sore nipples and other discomforts may be plaguing you as you adjust to this new routine.

Recovering after Caesarean

When you've had a C-section you're recovering from major surgery and need to treat yourself accordingly. Sleep when baby sleeps and stay away from strenuous activity and heavy lifting (nothing bigger than baby as a general rule). Use a bed pillow or a nursing pillow to hold your baby without pressuring your incision. Pain medication may be prescribed; if you're breastfeeding talk to your doctor about judicious use.

································· **need to know** ·························

Your doctor will recommend six weeks of rest and recuperation (within limits—you are a new mom after all), and you'll be advised not to drive while taking pain medications.

Second or subsequent C-section moms may recover a bit quicker, just because they know what to expect and treat themselves accordingly. Above all, don't push it, or you'll set your recovery back even further.

Baby's Body: An Operator's Manual

Your baby will actually lose weight as she starts out in life but should be back up to birth weight by her two-week checkup. Thereafter, she may put on one pound every two weeks, doubling her birth weight by month 4. Premature babies sometimes grow a little slower, but most will eventually catch up.

Her eyesight is a bit hazy, but she can see you fairly clearly when you hold her 7 to 10 inches away from your face. Studies show she knows your voice well already from listening to it in the womb and prefers it to a stranger's. Your newborn arrives with a variety of natural reflexes or involuntary ways of moving:

Palmar, or grasping, reflex. When you touch your baby's open hand, she'll make a fist around your finger.

Rooting reflex. If you stroke her cheek, her head will turn toward your touch. This reflex helps the bleary-eyed newborn find her food source, and you can use it to guide her to the breast or bottle.

Sucking reflex. Once at the breast or bottle, baby's sucking reflex takes over as she automatically sucks on anything put in her mouth.

Startle, or moro, reflex. When baby is startled, he will thrust his arms and legs out and arch his back, then quickly pull arms and legs in again.

Babinski reflex. Stroking baby's foot will make him spread his toes and flex his foot in.

Stepping reflex. Hold your baby up with your hands under her armpits so that her feet are touching a firm surface. She will lift her feet up and down like she is about to take baby steps.

Tonic neck reflex. When placed on his back, baby turns his head to the right and makes fists with his hands.

Blinking. The involuntary reflex of closing her eyes when they are exposed to bright light, air, or another stimulus is the one reflex that baby will keep for the rest of her life.

From Soft Spot to Curled Toes

The bones of baby's skull are not yet fused together, and unless you had a caesarean delivery your baby's head may look a bit, well, pointy. This cone-headed appearance is the result of pressure in the birth canal and will round out within a few weeks. There are four small areas on your baby's head where the baby's skull bones have not yet joined together, called fontanelles (or soft spots). Three of these fontanelles fuse within the first four months of life, but the longest lasting and most visible of these—the diamond-shaped area on the top of the head called the anterior fontanelle (or soft spot)—may take up to eighteen months to close. Many a curious sibling has reached out to jab this pulsating spot, much to their parent's horror. Don't get too concerned—your baby's brain is well protected by a tough membrane called the dura mater.

The eye color your baby has at birth may change later in infancy or childhood. This is due to the ongoing production of the hormone melanin, which can cause later eye color changes.

Baby's Skin

Your newborn's soft-as-butter skin may have some imperfections at first. Postterm babies are more likely to have some peeling, while preterm babies may still be sporting a substantial amount of lanugo and vernix. Although the vernix is fairly well rubbed off by the time you bring baby home, you may continue to find it in his creases and crevices until his first real bath. The lanugo will rub itself off over the next few weeks.

Baby may also be wearing one or more birthmarks on his birthday suit. Red marks on the eyelids, forehead, and at the very back of the nape of the neck usually fade and disappear over time and are called salmon patches or stork bites. Red, strawberry birthmarks can increase in size but may shrink and be gone by age five. Your baby may also have one or more light brown birthmarks known as café au lait spots. Very rarely, café au lait spots (particularly a large number of marks) are symptomatic of one of several uncommon medical conditions. Talk to your child's doctor if you have any concerns. Dark blue to blue-green spots on the buttocks or lower back are known as Mongolian spots. They are most common in African-American, Native American, and Asian newborns and fade over time. If your baby is born with what is known as a port wine stain, a bright red or purple mark that is considered to be more permanent, plastic surgery is an option in later life if they are located in a prominent spot. Ask your pediatrician or family doctor for more information.

Little whiteheads called milia are common on newborns, and you may see them around the nose. Caused by oil-secreting glands, the pimples may come and go during the first few days.

You may also see petechia, red to purple pinpoints, on baby's face from the trauma of coming down the birth canal. These will disappear in a few days as well.

The Umbilical Cord

Baby's umbilical cord stump looks just like it sounds, a dark, dried up protrusion. Since it is basically dead tissue, it is black in color. You'll be instructed to clean it regularly, usually with alcohol swabs, and keep it dry to prevent breakage and bleeding. Keep an eye open for signs of infection, such as pus or inflammation. Within two weeks or so, the stump will fall off and your baby's perfect little belly button will be revealed.

Genitals

Before your husband congratulates himself too heartily on your well-endowed son, you may want to break the news that it is probably just a passing phenomenon. Newborn boys and girls are often born with swollen genitals, again due to the effects of your pregnancy hormones working on them. Girls may even have a bit of mucus discharge, possibly blood-tinged, from their vaginas.

Fingernails and Toenails

Baby's tiny curled fingers and toes usually emerge in need of a manicure. Growing for several months in the womb, they are typically long and ragged. The thought of trimming such tiny appendages may fill you with dread, but it's not as hard as you might think. Just make sure you have the right tools (infant-sized clippers) and try to trim while baby is sleeping if you'd like to avoid wrestling with a moving target. If you still can't seem to get it down, bring your clippers with you to your two-week pediatrician appointment and ask for pointers.

Sleeping Like a Baby

In the beginning, it will seem like your little one is sleeping a lot. In fact, she's snoozing up to eighteen hours a day. If she's your first, you may be waiting to run in and get some quality playtime at the first rustle. While her sleep patterns, which involve four-hour stretches of snoozing, won't have a huge effect on your day schedule, they're going to hit you hard at night. She'll be waking up several times an evening for at least the first three months to be fed.

> ### need to know
>
> Baby should always be put to sleep on his back. If a thin blanket is necessary, place baby with his feet at the bottom end of the crib and make sure the blanket is tucked in between mattress and crib and goes no higher than baby's chest.

Remember to always place your baby on his back when laying him down for a nap or bedtime. Back sleeping has been shown to reduce the incidence of sudden infant death syndrome, or SIDS. Make sure baby's crib is clear of stuffed animals, quilts, pillows, and other soft bedding when he heads to bed as well.

Postpartum Depression

Feeling down is a common postpartum emotion that typically passes in a few weeks. For many women, however, these feelings go beyond the basic baby blues and signal a more serious depressive or endocrine disorder.

The Baby Blues

The majority of new mothers experience what has commonly become known as "the baby blues," a short-lived period of mild depression that appears in up to 85 percent of postpartum women. A severe shortage of sleep, disappointment with the birth experience, see-sawing hormone levels, anxieties about baby's health and well-being, and shaky confidence in your own parenting skills can all lead to feelings of sadness and inadequacy. Fortunately, most cases of the blues resolve themselves within a few days to two weeks after birth as balance returns to the new mother's life.

When It's More Than the Blues

More serious is postpartum depression (PPD), which occurs in about 10 percent of new mothers, and can drag on for up to a year. If you're experiencing one or more of the following symptoms, talk to your doctor about PPD:

- Feelings of extreme sadness and inexplicable crying jags
- Lack of pleasure in things you would normally enjoy
- Trouble concentrating
- Excessive worrying, or conversely, a lack of interest in the baby
- Feelings of low self-esteem
- Decreased appetite

Fortunately, PPD can be effectively treated with counseling and/or antidepressant drugs, so ask your doctor for a referral to a mental health professional. Even if you're breastfeeding, you may have medication options; there are several antidepressant drugs on the market that are thought to have minimal effects on nursing infants. A number of studies involving sertraline (Zoloft), for example, found that while the drug passes into breastmilk, the levels it reaches in the nursing infant were clinically insignificant, in some cases too low to even be detected in standard laboratory blood tests. Safety cannot be guaranteed, however; studies on how antidepressants might affect a breastfed child in the long term are not available. On the other hand, clinical research has demonstrated a measurable detrimental effect on children of depressed mothers when PPD goes untreated. Each woman must evaluate the risks of treatment versus the benefits when deciding if drug therapy is right for them.

Postpartum Psychosis

One in every 1,000 women experiences a severe form of PPD known as postpartum psychosis (or puerperal psychosis). Symptoms include hallucinations, delusions, contemplation of hurting oneself or others, insomnia, and turbulent mood swings. Postpartum psychosis is a medical emergency that needs immediate treatment and usually hospitalization. The good news is with proper medical care full recovery is expected.

Thyroid Problems

Thyroid problems are fairly common after childbirth, but the symptoms can be confused with other postpartum conditions. Milk supply difficulties, extreme fatigue, hair loss, depression, mood changes, problems losing weight or unusually rapid weight loss, heart palpitations, menstrual irregularities, and sleep disorders are all common signs of postpartum thyroid conditions.

.... **need to know** ....

Some women have temporary postpartum hyperthyroidism—an overactive thyroid, with weight loss, diarrhea, racing heart, anxiety, and other symptoms of a revved up metabolism.

Doctors may prescribe drugs to ease symptoms, but this condition often resolves itself quickly. Other women can develop temporary postpartum hypothyroidism—an underactive thyroid—with fatigue, weight gain, constipation, depression, and other symptoms of a slowed-down metabolism. Again, medication may be prescribed, depending on the severity of symptoms, and frequently the thyroid will return to normal within six months to a year after the birth. New mothers with a family or personal history of autoimmune or thyroid disease may benefit from routine thyroid testing in the first month postpartum. It can be hard to tell what's "normal" after having a baby, but if any of the above symptoms become debilitating, a thyroid test can quickly rule out or diagnose a thyroid problem. Women who experience temporary postpartum thyroid problems are at a higher risk to develop thyroid disease later in life and should talk to their doctor about regular followup screening.

Adjusting to Your New Schedule

Many aspects of your life will be different now that you are a parent. You will probably feel that your priorities are very different now that you have a little one to think about. But taking time to care for yourself is equally important.

Sleep, or Lack of It

People told you how tired you would be when baby arrived, but after three months of uncomfortable and interrupted sleep leading up to the delivery, you thought you were well prepared. Surprise. You feel like the walking dead and crave sleep constantly. Your baby will sleep through the night eventually. In the meantime, give yourself a break by splitting night duties with your spouse or significant others. Even if you're breastfeeding, if baby is in another room he can help out by retrieving and returning him. Also remember the new mom credo: "Nap when the baby naps." Forget laundry, forget dishes. You need your rest more than a clean house right now. And if you've only slept three hours last night between bouts of calming a fussy baby? Don't get behind the wheel of a car before you get some adequate shut-eye. Extreme fatigue slows your reaction time and you run a very real risk of falling asleep behind the wheel.

Don't Forget to Have Fun

Once you get past the fatigue, the uncertainties, and the occasional frustrations, being a new mom can be incredibly entertaining.

You have a legitimate excuse to play, explore, rhyme, sing, and revisit your childhood in general. You have an adoring little person who hangs on your every word and movement and loves you unconditionally. And you get to witness all her incredible firsts as your tiny miracle learns to smile, roll over, crawl, and eventually walk and talk. In a year, this postpartum time will be a distant memory. Treasure it while it's here.

The Rest of the Family

Obviously, you aren't doing this alone. Even if you're a single mom, you have people in your life who care for you and baby. Involve your family, or those around you, and baby and you will benefit.

Support

You might learn that your mother really does know a thing or two. It's amazing to watch her, and your dad, soothe and burp their grandchild like they were just doing it yesterday. They often have a baby wrangling trick or two up their sleeve that will make your life easier. Every family relationship is different, of course, but witnessing someone who raised you cuddle and care for the child that you now nurture instills a sense of connectivity and completeness, as if your life has come full circle. Now just hope that all those prophecies they made about "hoping you have a child just like you" don't come to fruition! Neighbors and friends will likely call to both check on the new addition and find out if they can do anything for you. One simple rule: take all help that is offered. Don't feel guilty. They wouldn't offer if they didn't mean it. And if they offered just because they thought they should, they'll think twice next time won't they?

Sibling Rivalry

Give your older child a chance to bond with baby on the sibling level as well. Older kids frequently get a kick out of holding, feeding, and "protecting" their new little sister or brother. Children who are preschool age or younger may have a more difficult time accepting this drain on their parents' attention. Some tips to promote sibling harmony:

- If you're breastfeeding, establish a family routine of a snack or story when baby nurses to make it a special time for all.

- Involve your child in age-appropriate baby care. Helping with a bath or diaper change may be just the incentive they need to relish their new big brother or sister role.

- Try to arrange some special parental one-on-one time. Even if it's just a quick story during baby's nap, try to have a designated time where your firstborn is the star of the show.

- Tell your older child stories about their babyhood. Hearing how they threw strained peas at daddy or wore their very ripe diaper as a hat will have them in stitches and may help them relate to this odd little creature a bit better.

- Don't use the baby as an excuse. If they hear "We can't do that because the baby is sleeping" constantly, guess who they will start to blame for the new crimp in their social life? Instead, provide baby-friendly alternatives when you say no: "We can't go swimming today, but we can go for a walk to the park." And arrange some time to take your "big kid" someplace he's been dying to go without a sibling in tow.

Daddy Time

Don't hog the baby. Make sure that daddy gets his own chance at bonding time. With a constant flow of visitors and your many hours clocked on baby duty, he may be feeling left out. Both he and your child need time alone together. Getting out and moving for a short walk is good exercise for you right now and a good way to clear your head after a day of talking in babyspeak. Hand the reins over, without direction or judgment if at all possible, and give dad a chance to run the show.

Chapter 17

Your New Life

Although it seems overwhelming at first, it won't take you long to get the parenting basics down. Making career and family choices, building new and stronger relationships with your partner, and getting back in tune with your body are all priorities during the first year postpartum.

Getting Your Body Back

Another time-worn motherhood maxim that is worth repeating: It took nine months for you to look this way, so give yourself at least that much time to get your body back. Actually, giving yourself a year is perhaps more realistic if you factor in a three-month transitional period after the birth of your child. As you hammer out a routine where you and baby can manage to get dressed and bathed before dinnertime, you won't have much time for structured exercise in those early days.

In general, most women need to lose about ten more pounds to return to their prepregnant weight at their six-week postpartum visit. Many women find it difficult to lose weight during this period because they're working hard, nursing, and sleep-deprived. The time crunch all new mothers face can make a sensible and nutritious diet and regular exercise seem like a monumental task. Start slow and easy and the rest will follow.

The Incredible Changing Baby

Your infant will reach new milestones in such dizzying succession that you'll be convinced you have a prodigy on your hands. Watch her transform from a floppy-necked, bleary-eyed newborn to an active and alert infant in a matter of months. As she starts to become more aware of her surroundings, and interact more with you and her environment, providing encouragement, stimulation, and patience will help her to thrive.

Your pediatrician will give you an idea of appropriate developmental milestones as your baby grows.

your new life

The main function of milestones are to serve as a screening tool; if baby is lagging on many it may be a sign of a problem, but one or more delays are typically no cause for concern.

A Whole New Family

Beyond your new parenting relationship, other family dynamics have definitely changed since baby's arrival. You and your partner may find yourselves hard pressed for time to spend together, and practical matters like money may be more of an issue as you learn how to adjust your lifestyle and income for three (or more). If you have some specific goals for family planning, you may even be thinking about pregnancy again.

Intimacy Issues

Perhaps for the first time in months, you may be rediscovering your interest in sex. Of course, your little one may be putting a damper on things unwittingly—rest assured she is bound to interrupt you in the height of passion at least once. Flexibility is key in having a healthy sex life with kids around. Grab time together when it presents itself, and follow the following tips for rekindling the fire.

- **No baby talk.** Calling each other mommy and daddy around the kids is fine, but it can really kill the mood if it slips out in other circumstances.
- **Take it slow and easy.** Give both of you time to rediscover each other. There may be a learning curve with your postpregnancy body.

- **Love yourself.** It's hard to enjoy lovemaking if you're self-conscious about the way you look. Accept the state of your body, whatever it is, and see it instead as a visible symbol of the miracle of your baby.
- **Quiet please.** You don't need to turn the baby monitor up to eleven. Hearing every tiny baby sigh is a turnoff. Just turn the monitor down, or open your door instead; if she wakes up she will let you know.

Financial Planning

By now you've gotten a feel of how much it costs to care for your new family member, and you're either pleasantly surprised or in a panic. If it's the former, pat yourself on the back and consider saving your extra pennies in a new college fund for your child (a financial advisor can help you explore your options). If you're in the panic category, take a deep breath and try to pinpoint the problem. Are the extra expenses coming from baby gadgetry and other nonessential purchases, or from necessities like diapers and wipes? A budget is really important in assessing the family finances now, so if you didn't create one during pregnancy, now is the time to start. There are places to cut back if you look for them. Finally, if you find yourself hopelessly in debt no matter how you look at the situation, you need to see a reputable credit counselor to get back on your financial footing.

The Next Time Around

The first birthday is usually about the time when everyone starts asking about a brother or sister for your "big'" kid. When you're done rolling your eyes and laughing, you start to actually give it some serious consideration. Are you ready to do it all over again? Beyond physical readiness, how will you know? Suddenly, the sight of another woman in her ninth month brings about warm memories instead of enormous relief that it's someone else and not you, and you seem to have all but forgotten the perils of pregnancy and pain of childbirth. If you're sold on a family with kids close enough in age to play and go to the same school together, you may be ready to start a bit sooner.

---

need to know

Try to give your body time to recover so that you don't cheat yourself and your next child out of a healthy pregnancy. A two-year breather from birth to birth is ideal.

Losing any excess pounds before starting over will make it easier for you to get through and beyond the next pregnancy.

Index